I've hea   *... Is that true?*

How can I tell if I have a cold, a flu, sinusitis, an allergy—or something else?

Should I exercise when I have a cold?

Which over-the-counter cold remedies are best avoided?

For all its wizardry, modern science can't yet provide us with a cure for the common cold. But there *are* ways of reducing your risk of catching a cold—and keeping the sneezing and sniffling to a minimum if you do catch one.

This guide takes you through the maze of conflicting advice and explains how simple, natural techniques can help you prevent and combat colds and flu. Using the best of both conventional and alternative medicine, this is the book that can help *you* win the cold war!

THE NATURAL WAY TO BEAT
THE COMMON COLD AND FLU

*A Holistic Approach
for Prevention and Relief*

RICHARD TRUBO

Richard Trubo

BERKLEY BOOKS, NEW YORK

NOTICE: This book is intended as a reference volume only, not as a medical manual. The information here is designed to help you make informed decisions about your health. It is not a substitute for any treatment that may have been prescribed by your doctor. If you suspect that you have a medical problem, we urge you to seek competent medical help.

THE NATURAL WAY TO BEAT THE COMMON COLD AND FLU

A Berkley Book / published by arrangement with
the author

PRINTING HISTORY
Berkley edition / November 1998

All rights reserved.
Copyright © 1998 by Richard Trubo.
Book design by Casey Hampton.
This book may not be reproduced in whole or in part,
by mimeograph or any other means, without permission.
For information address:
The Berkley Publishing Group, a member of Penguin Putnam Inc.,
375 Hudson Street, New York, New York 10014.

The Penguin Putnam Inc. World Wide Web site address is
http://www.penguinputnam.com

ISBN: 0-425-16625-2

BERKLEY®
Berkley Books are published by The Berkley Publishing Group,
a member of Penguin Putnam Inc.,
375 Hudson Street, New York, New York 10014.
BERKLEY and the "B" design
are trademarks belonging to Berkley Publishing Corporation.

PRINTED IN THE UNITED STATES OF AMERICA

10 9 8 7 6 5 4 3 2 1

CONTENTS

ACKNOWLEDGMENTS

Thanks to Denise Silvestro for her valuable editorial support and for making this project possible; and to Jane Dystel for her unwavering guidance and expertise as an agent on my behalf.

Thanks to the doctors and scientists who shared their clinical experiences and research findings—most notably, Gustav Belz, John Bogden, David Bresler, Barrie Cassilith, James Duke, John Heinerman, Steven Mostow, Isadore Rosenfeld, Martin Rossman, Victor Sierpina, Art Ulene, and George Ulett.

THE NATURAL WAY TO BEAT THE COMMON COLD AND FLU

1

A Billion Colds a Year!

*There is just one way to treat the common cold—
with contempt!*

—Sir William Osler
Johns Hopkins University physician

Every year, at the first sneeze of winter, it seems to
happen all over again. Your throat becomes scratchy.
Your head feels stuffy and your eyes are watery. The
floodgates of your nose burst open, and the chills leave
you shaking and shivering from head to toe. You feel
like doing nothing but crawling into bed, turning up the
electric blanket to 10, cuddling up with a bottle of vitamin C, and hibernating for the next 72 hours. Sure,
you could race off to your doctor's office, but you know
exactly what you have. Welcome to another clash with
the common cold.

If you're like most people, you're probably assaulted
by colds several times a year—and it doesn't seem fair.
After all, in this era of medical miracles—when cutting-
edge drugs and high-tech diagnostic tests are the norm—
the common cold stubbornly perseveres. During the
height of the cold season, everyone around you seems
to be sneezing, and cold viruses lurk just about every-

where, from subway turnstiles to elevator buttons. No wonder you might feel that your chances of remaining sniffle-free are about as promising as those of winning the state lottery.

But instead of barricading yourself indoors, protected by a fortress of tissue and cold medications, it may be time to examine your other options for winning the cold wars. By taking a holistic approach—using the best of both conventional and alternative medicine—you may be able to keep your distance from the pesky bugs that yearn to cause trouble. Even when colds do strike, you can soften their assault and get back on your feet more quickly by relying on natural treatments, along with what your doctor has to offer. With a few key lifestyle changes, and a willingness to explore options such as vitamins, minerals, herbs, and homeopathy, you can improve your chances of staying healthy during the cold season, while those around you have their handkerchiefs and humidifiers at the ready.

THE COLD FACTS

The common cold couldn't be more common. This inflammation of the upper respiratory tract afflicts the average adult two to four times a year, and children about six to eight times a year. Women appear more susceptible than men, perhaps because they are surrounded more often by sniffling and coughing children. Youngsters are more likely to fall prey to cold viruses than adults, simply because their immune systems are still maturing, and they're often in close contact with sneezing peers in day-care centers and classrooms.

Here are the people at greatest risk of catching colds:

- Infants and young children up to the age of 6
- Parents with young children
- Smokers
- People with weakened immune systems
- Members of low-income families (who tend to live in crowded conditions)
- People under stress
- People who don't exercise

Although colds can certainly make you miserable, they are usually more of a nuisance than anything else. Yes, they can leave you saying uncle as you struggle with a drippy or congested nose; plenty of sneezing; a sore throat; sinus discomfort; a headache; a dry, hacking cough; and perhaps a low-grade fever (usually under 100 degrees). The infection, typically localized in the upper respiratory tract (from the nostrils to the throat), can linger for about seven to ten days, but once the symptoms have run their course, they're gone for good—until the next cold appears.

In the meantime, more people visit their doctors' offices with colds than with any other ailment. Americans endure a staggering *one billion* colds a year, and in the process, the average person misses about seven days of work annually due to the sniffles. That's certainly nothing to sneeze at.

THE VIRULENT VIRUSES

So what's to blame for all of those runny noses? The culprits are tiny, submicroscopic viruses that trigger the disease process—about 200 different viral strains in all. The most common of these viruses are from a family called *rhinoviruses* (from the Greek word *rhin,* meaning "nose"); they are responsible for about 20 to 40 percent of colds in adults. *Coronaviruses* account for another 10 to 15 percent of colds; the remainder include influenza, parainfluenza, RSV (respiratory syncytial virus), and enterovirus. Most common in the winter and early spring, these organisms enter the body through the nose and the eyes, and then settle into the mucous membranes of the nose or attach themselves to cells in the throat; the temperatures of these friendly environments hover above 90 degrees, which is conducive to rapid viral proliferation. The body tries to fight back by dispatching white blood cells to the site of the infection. But too often, the cold virus packs the wallop of Muhammad Ali's hook in his prime, and it overwhelms the body's defenders. After an incubation period, usually one to two days, you may find yourself sneezing and sniffling for a week to ten days.

Where are you most likely to contract these viruses? You might get nervous riding in a crowded elevator next to someone who's blowing his nose, or sitting in an office cubicle with co-workers who are hacking and coughing. But while germ-laden droplets from these kinds of sneezes and coughs can certainly spread the cold virus, they aren't the primary means of transmission, says infectious-diseases specialist Steven Mostow, M.D., of Columbia Rose Medical Center in Denver. In fact, direct and indirect hand-to-hand transmission is more the rule than the exception. Shake hands with someone with a cold, and you could pick up the cold virus. Turn a doorknob just touched by a cold sufferer, and you might find yourself sneezing in a day or two. The virus could be lying in wait on telephones, handrails, pens, and coffeepot handles, and once it's transmitted to your hands, you could set the disease process into motion with a simple touch of your nose or eyes. Research by Jack Gwaltney, Jr., M.D., and his colleagues at the University of Virginia in Charlottesville has concluded that when people touch their noses and eyes with virus-contaminated droplets, nearly three-quarters of them catch colds.

What's the most contagious time for viral transmission? Once you're infected, you're most likely to spread the virus beginning about 24 hours *before* you start to sneeze and cough, and then during the first day or two after symptoms appear.

Kissing: Safer Than You Think?

Just because your spouse or lover has a cold, that's not necessarily a reason to set up a Berlin Wall–like barrier between the two of you. In fact, kissing is not a common way of catching a cold.

At the Common Cold Unit in Salisbury, England, researchers examined the routes by which colds are most easily transmitted. When it was introduced into the noses of volunteers, about one-third of them developed a cold. When the virus was placed in their mouths and throats, however, none became sick. The conclusion: You may be quite safe kissing someone with a cold!

Come In from the Rain?

When you were a kid, your mother might have cautioned you to avoid drafts, dress warmly during cold weather, and stay indoors when you had wet hair—all to keep colds at bay. But the common-cold experts have quite another message, insisting that none of those strategies really matters. Colds are caused by viruses, they say, not by dampness, drafts, the chills, or a falling thermometer. That's a scientific fact. In an experiment in England in the late 1940s, volunteers were divided into three groups: One group was exposed to a dose of cold virus; another received no virus, but stood in a draft in wet bathing suits for 30 minutes; and the final group was exposed to both the virus and the chilly environment. The results? The virus was the real mischief-maker. In fact, chilling alone did not produce a single cold, even when the experiments were repeated.

Of course, evidence like this raises the inevitable question: "Why are colds more common in the fall and winter, when you're more likely to be blasted by wet weather and chilly temperatures?" Researchers at the National Institute of Allergy and Infectious Diseases believe that the answer rests with the increased amount of time that we spend indoors in the colder months. People are more likely to catch cold viruses in an enclosed environment in close proximity to someone who is already sick. Also, the lower humidity of winter is more conducive to viral proliferation; at the same time, central heating systems tend to dry out the mucous membranes of the nasal passages, increasing their likelihood of attracting viruses. No wonder it's the cold-weather months when you're more likely to become as congested as a New York subway train at rush hour.

IS THE FLU LEAVING YOU BLUE?

Like it or not, during virtually every fall and winter, the flu (also called *influenza*) is headed to a neighborhood near you. Like the common cold, it is a respiratory infection caused by a virus. Even though the flu tends to be a more malevolent illness, some of its symptoms (runny nose, cough) are deceptively coldlike; for that reason, the flu is sometimes misdiagnosed as a severe cold.

Flu season typically begins in November or December, and lingers through March and April. In a typical year, the flu afflicts about 10 to 20 percent of the population, but in the worst outbreaks, it is much more widespread and can even become a killer. The 1918–1919 pandemic of the Spanish flu killed 20 million people worldwide (see the box on page 8). Today, in an average year, about 10,000 to 20,000 Americans die from the flu and its complications (usually pneumonia).

The Spanish Flu Pandemic

In 1918 and 1919, as World War I was drawing to a close, a vicious influenza pandemic spread around the globe. Its toll in the United States and other countries was staggering. Half of the world's population was stricken with the flu, and 20 million people lost their lives to it before it finally ran its course. It not only assaulted the very young and the very old, whose immune systems may have been weaker because of their ages, but it also killed many adults in their twenties and thirties (scientists have never determined why the pandemic claimed the lives of so many young adults).

In the United States, not only did about 500,000 people die from this so-called Spanish flu, but during its height, most Americans were forced to make changes in their day-to-day lives. Many schools closed temporarily in hopes of stopping the spread of the disease. Other places where people came together—including churches and movie houses—shut down as well. In New York City, the health commissioner insisted that people cover their mouths and noses with a handkerchief whenever they sneezed. At Navy bases, blowtorches were used hourly to sterilize drinking fountains. In Philadelphia, the city's only morgue couldn't handle all of the bodies of people who had fallen victim to influenza; at one point, corpses were piled atop one another in every unused room (even in the hallways).

By the time the pandemic had run its course, the casualties left in its wake were five times higher than

the number of Americans who had died on the battle-
fields in World War I. Subsequent epidemics have
taken ominous tolls as well—for instance, the 1957–
1958 ''Asian flu'' caused 70,000 deaths in the United
States, and the 1968–1969 ''Hong Kong flu'' claimed
another 34,000 lives. But nothing in recent history
has ever compared to the nightmare perpetuated by
the Spanish flu.

What Causes the Flu?

Back in the fourteenth century in Italy, an unusual align-
ment of the planets was believed to *influenze* the development of what came to be known as influenza. Today,
we know that the cause of the flu is found not in the
stars, but rather in viruses. Although about 200 viruses
can cause the common cold, the flu is associated with
just three viral types, called influenza A, B, and C.

Most severe flu outbreaks are caused by the type A
virus, while type B is responsible for milder cases. The
type C virus can produce symptoms that are typically no
more serious than those of the common cold. However,
because these viruses can *mutate*, or change themselves,
from one flu season to the next—altering their surface
proteins and thus creating new viral strains—your body
really doesn't build up immunity to the flu, and must
fight the good fight against it year after year.

The flu tends to be highly contagious—even more
contagious than the common cold. It's likely to be
passed from one person to another through coughs,
transported on airborne droplets. The influenza virus can
also be transmitted when an infected person touches
someone else. In confined spaces, the flu virus can wreak

havoc; in 1977, for example, doctors traced a flu outbreak in Kodiak, Alaska, to a single flu-infected woman
traveling in a commercial jet; as the air in the plane
recirculated again and again, 38 of the 54 passengers
contracted the disease, and in turn spread it to many
friends and family members in the ensuing days.

Is the "Stomach Flu" Really the Flu?

As everyday illnesses go, the ''stomach flu'' is rather
hideous. It can cause an upset stomach, abdominal
cramps, diarrhea, nausea, and vomiting. Not much
fun. Just ask George Bush, who was blindsided by
the stomach flu when he visited Tokyo in 1992 and
threw up on his Japanese host at a state dinner—and
then collapsed. Emily Post would have been horri-
fied!

Although the terms *stomach flu* and *intestinal flu*
(as well as *traveler's diarrhea*) are commonly attached to this disorder, it really isn't the flu at all.
Influenza, after all, is a respiratory infection. That's
why doctors use the word *gastroenteritis* to describe
these acute infections of the stomach and intestines,
which are caused by a variety of microorganisms
(such as rotavirus, *Escherichia coli,* and *Salmonella*
bacteria). The treatment usually includes rest and
drinking plenty of fluids to replace what is lost
through diarrhea.

Do You Have the Flu?

The common cold can make you miserable. But the flu can leave you feeling as though you've been ravaged by an 8.8 earthquake and dozens of aftershocks. Although you can harbor the influenza virus for one to three days before symptoms first appear, once they show their colors, you'll know it. If you've got a raging fever (over 101 degrees), if you have the chills one minute and are drenched with perspiration the next, if your throbbing headache feels as if your skull is going to burst, if you're coughing up a storm and can barely swallow, if you're as achy and fatigued as if you had just run a marathon— you've probably been flattened by the flu. Although you might be able to work at your desk with a cold, influenza can leave you begging for mercy and pleading for a few days of R&R to recover. Even after the symptoms subside, typically after seven to fourteen days, you might feel weary and worn for weeks.

While it's hard to imagine having the flu and not realizing it, some of the symptoms associated with colds, flu, and allergies overlap, and that can sometimes cause confusion. Certain allergies, in fact, can become worse during the cold and flu season, as people spend more time indoors during the winter months and are exposed for greater periods of time to dust mites, pet dander, household molds, and other triggers of allergy-related runny noses and coughs. The chart on the next page will help you sort out which disorder you actually have.

What's Bothering You: Allergy, Cold, or Flu?

	Allergy	Common Cold	Flu
Runny/ stuffy nose	common	common	sometimes
Fever	never	low-grade	high
Headache	rare	rare	prominent
Sore throat	sometimes	common	sometimes
Sneezing	common	common	sometimes
Cough	sometimes	mild	common
Itchy eyes/ nose	common	rare	rare
Aches and pains	never	slight	severe
Fatigue	rare	mild	severe, persistent

A PLAN OF ACTION

Over the years, many of the remedies suggested for colds and flus were, by today's standards, rather mind-boggling. England's Common Cold Unit has collected these recommendations, which ranged from having patients sniff pepper or cinnamon to encouraging them to wash out their noses with cod liver oil. Cold sufferers were once advised to rub their socks with onions, avoid salads, tie cucumber slices to their ankles, eat red-pepper sandwiches, grow a moustache, wear a gas mask, or stand naked in front of an electric fan—all in the name of good health.

Fortunately, today's treatments have a stronger scientific grounding, although there is still controversy surrounding some of them. There are not yet any miracle cures or magic bullets, but plenty of reasonable strategies, both inside and outside mainstream medicine, can reduce the number of colds you get, and help you manage those that have blasted their way through. With pharmaceutical companies looking for new drugs to ease symptoms, and with the federal government's Office of Alternative Medicine funding research into an array of unconventional and complementary therapies, people now have more options than ever before. That's what this book is about. The information in the following pages will help you prevent colds and navigate successfully through the flood and fury of cold and flu symptoms, and make yourself more comfortable in the process.

2

Eating Smart: Diet Makes a Difference

What's one of the best weapons in your personal germ warfare against the common cold? Eating properly is an excellent foundation for staying cold-free or for making a more rapid recovery.

It sounds simple, doesn't it? Maybe too simple. But your diet can give your infection-fighting immune system a shot in the arm (and everywhere else), meal after meal. And that can help keep cold and flu viruses in hiding.

Let's start with a brief physiology lesson. The immune system is a complex matrix of specialized white blood cells (such as T-lymphocytes), proteins, and antibodies. Their collective job is to devour any and all foreign substances that invade the body. However, the immune system can weaken, and thus you often must rely on every tool at your disposal to keep it strong and vigilant, whether you're young or old.

"Many people experience declines in their immune

system with aging, but it isn't inevitable," says John Bogden, Ph.D., professor of preventive medicine and community health at the University of Medicine and Dentistry of New Jersey (UMDNJ). "In fact, after the age of 50, only about one-third of the population experiences this decline." Nevertheless, even young adult volunteers have developed compromised immunity when their diets had just mild deficiencies in nutrients such as vitamins A, B_6, C, and E and folic acid. Studies show that if you're not getting enough of even a single nutrient, your immune system can become impaired and you'll have an increased risk of illness.

So to stay cold-free, keep your focus on food. Eat smart, with an emphasis on plenty of vegetables, fruits, whole grains, and low-fat dairy products. They will help keep your resistance high, and vanquish the viruses trying to vandalize your body.

VEGGING OUT

Some of the best nutritional advice is also the most basic and mundane: When it comes to diet, start by consuming plenty of veggies. Produce is an excellent source of not only crucial vitamins, but also many so-called phytochemicals (*phyto* is a Greek word meaning "plant") that help overpower disease. These phytochemicals can function as *antioxidants* (substances that protect cells from damage) and appear to interfere with and even reverse declines in immune function.

Kenneth Cooper, M.D., the guru of aerobic exercise, advises consuming plenty of antioxidant-rich foods and supplements (bursting with vitamins C and E and beta-carotene) to fight off viruses and boost your defenses against the common cold. In up to nine servings a day, you'll be getting plenty of vitamin C, for example, which is a crucial player in the functioning of the immune system. Vitamin C stimulates the body's production of antibodies that can run roughshod over infectious agents. Studies show that if you're also consuming plenty of vitamin A–rich foods—such as carrots, sweet potatoes, turnip greens, and peppers—you'll maintain a robust immune system and improve your chances of ambushing cold bugs. Vitamin E, found in vegetable and seed oils (including soybean, sunflower, and cottonseed) and green leafy vegetables, can provide the knockout blow against disease-causing microorganisms.

Vitamin A and Beta-Carotene: Go to the Source

Vitamin A can increase the activity of your immune system, thus helping to trounce infectious viruses. Beta-carotene, the best studied of the carotenoids (precursors or building blocks of vitamin A), provides the pigment for many vegetables and fruits (it gives carrots their orange color; most foods rich in beta-carotene have deep orange, red, yellow, or green hues). More important, beta-carotene functions as an antioxidant, neutralizing toxic substances (called *free radicals*) produced in the body during normal metabolism, and destroying them before they can damage healthy cells.

To get plenty of vitamin A and beta-carotene, make sure that the following foods are a regular part of your diet (the richest sources of vitamin A and beta-carotene appear at the beginning of each list):

VITAMIN A

carrots	turnip	guavas
mangoes	greens	avocados
butternut	mustard	brussels sprouts
squash	greens	asparagus
Hubbard	Swiss chard	apricots
squash	tomatoes	prunes
vegetable soup	parsley	peaches
(chunky)	broccoli	
cantaloupe	nectarines	
kale	tangerines	
beet greens		

BETA-CAROTENE

carrots	sweet potatoes	romaine lettuce
collard	spinach	mangoes
greens	pink grapefruit	guavas
chicory leaf	mustard greens	broccoli
spinach	peaches	beet greens
cantaloupe	pumpkin	celery
winter	tomatoes	
squash	apricots	
kale		
red peppers		

Vitamin C: Citrus and Other Sources

While you probably think of orange juice as the best source of vitamin C, there are plenty of other excellent places to get it. Here are some of the richest dietary sources of vitamin C:

guavas	broccoli	honeydew melon
orange juice	tomato juice	green peas
sweet pepper	sweet potatoes	grapefruit
papayas	strawberries	cauliflower
oranges	potatoes	cantaloupe
mangoes	marinara sauce	brussels sprouts
kiwi	kale	butternut squash
grapefruit	lemons	acorn squash

Where to Get Your Vitamin E

Vitamin E is widely available in foods, although much of it is contained in fats and oils. If you're sticking to a low-fat diet, choose your food sources of vitamin E carefully. Here are common sources of vitamin E:

wheat-germ oil	wheat germ	safflower oil
corn oil	sweet potatoes	milk
soybean oil	sunflower oil	soybeans

macadamia	almond oil	lima beans
nuts	almonds	mangoes
hazelnuts	mayonnaise	peaches
cottonseed oil	apricots	olives
canola oil	asparagus	

THE CRUCIFEROUS CRUNCH

When you're choosing vegetables for your dinner plate, think cruciferous. These veggies, which include broccoli and cabbage, are particularly wondrous and potentially cold-crippling. They are probably best known as cancer fighters; they contain compounds called glucobrassicin, dithiolthiones, and benzyl isothiocyanate, which, once in the body, can shield you from several types of cancer. But they also can help bolster the immune system, thus helping fight infections. (See the adjoining box for a list of common cruciferous vegetables.)

A Plateful of Cruciferous Veggies

Cruciferous vegetables should be part of your daily diet, and not only because of their potential to boost your infection-fighting immune system. They also contain cancer-fighting chemicals that activate enzymes capable of transporting carcinogens (cancer-causing substances) away from the cells. The most common cruciferous veggies include the following:

bok choy	cauliflower	mustard greens
broccoli	collard greens	rutabaga
brussels sprouts	kale	turnip greens
cabbage	kohlrabi	turnips

MUSHROOM MADNESS

Mushrooms have risen to the top of the vegetable bin, thanks to their apparent antiviral and immunity-enhancing properties. In a study at the University of Michigan, researchers discovered in mushrooms an antiviral substance called lentinan, which appears capable of boosting immune function. In Asian countries, shiitake mushrooms are often prescribed for battling the common cold, as well as for improving blood circulation. Reishi mushrooms are sometimes recommended for people with low immunity; because reishis are not particularly appetizing, they're available in capsule form in health-food stores.

Feed a Cold? Or Starve It?

Certainly you've heard the old adage, "Feed a cold, starve a fever"—although some people insist that it's really "Feed a fever, starve a cold."

Actually, neither is a hard-and-fast rule. In fact, there's no evidence that either stuffing yourself or starving yourself is the magic formula that can deliver you from the sniffles.

Most doctors believe that in the midst of an illness, you should listen to your body and your appetite. If you feel like eating, then eat; your body can certainly use the calories during your recovery. But if food just doesn't appeal to you, then push the plate away (although it's probably not wise to stay *completely* away from food). Whatever the case, be sure to drink plenty of fluids, particularly if you have the flu and a fever (that's the time when your need for fluids increases); aim for at least six to eight glasses a day of hot or cold fluids to ensure that you don't fall prey to dehydration.

GARLIC GUSTO

In 1965, when an influenza epidemic swept through parts of the former Soviet Union, the government airlifted a 500-ton emergency shipment of raw garlic into hard-hit regions. Residents were advised to consume garlic because of its "qualities for preventing flu." That directive wasn't really anything new. Throughout history, garlic's medicinal properties have been highly touted. A large body of folklore has built up around garlic, including claims that wearing a clove around your neck can chase away witches and vampires. In recent years, garlic has been subjected to plenty of scientific scrutiny—more than a thousand studies have been published since the 1950s—and there is clearly more to the "stinking rose" than its offensive odor. Research shows that it can guard against heart disease by reducing cholesterol, activating clot-busting proteins, and reducing blood pressure; it can also interfere with the development of some types of cancer, including colon and stomach cancers.

But what about the common cold? In sniffing out the facts, scientists have carefully analyzed many of the 200-plus chemicals in garlic, and their attention has been drawn to a compound called *allicin*. This chemical forms when a garlic clove is cut or crushed, and its antiviral activity against colds and influenza has been demonstrated in laboratory experiments. At Brigham Young University, investigators have reported that garlic extract destroyed almost all of the rhinoviruses and influenza viruses to which it was exposed. However, even though research like this may be on the right track, remember that it's a giant leap from a test-tube experiment to the real world. Medical anthropologist John Heinerman, Ph.D., the author of *Nature's Super Seven Medicines*, says that the sulfur in garlic is the real hero, specifically because it boosts the production of macrophages in the immune network. "These macrophages are large, garbage-collecting cells—sort of the street sweepers of the immune system," scooping up the invading organisms that might be running rampant in your body, he says. So when you've got a cold, consuming garlic as part of a hot soup, for example, may be just what the doctor ordered.

How much garlic is enough? About one clove (4 grams) of garlic per day may be all that you need. But that could also be enough to send your friends running for cover, thanks to your garlic-ravaged breath. That's why many people are getting their garlic from supplements these days, popping capsules containing dried garlic powder. These pills can get allicin into your body without risking any friendships.

"I recommend to my own patients that they take the garlic tablets," says Gustav Belz, M.D., director of the Centre for Cardiovascular Pharmacology in Mainz, Germany. "Certainly from a social standpoint, it's more acceptable than eating cloves."

But not everyone is a pill proponent. "My opinion is that if it doesn't stink, it's not as good!" insists James Duke, Ph.D., a botanist with a 30-year career at the U.S. Department of Agriculture. Dr. Duke sticks to raw garlic unless he's going to be in the company of people; then, he resorts to capsules. A typical dose when you're struggling with a cold is two capsules a day, he says.

Even at high doses, garlic doesn't seem to present any significant downside. Occasionally, people have allergic reactions to the odoriferous bulb, causing conditions such as dermatitis. But the risks are minimal. "There are centuries of experience with garlic, so we'd know about anything really harmful if it existed," says Dr. Belz. "Garlic is extremely well tolerated."

SAY YES TO YOGURT

You probably think of those containers of yogurt in your refrigerator as a tasty low-fat snack. But they are actually much more. They also can provide a boost to your immune function, and thus help put a cap on colds and the flu.

Yogurt is essentially milk that has been fermented by

adding bacteria to it. As with garlic, a rich folklore surrounds yogurt, including claims that it can prolong life. Decades ago, in fact, a Russian researcher claimed that a 100-year-old man's longevity could be credited primarily to his consumption of yogurt.

A study at the University of California, Davis, put yogurt to the test. One group of volunteers consumed two cups of low-fat, live active yogurt a day; others ate the same amount of yogurt, but without the live active cultures; a final group ate no yogurt.

After four months, investigators studied blood samples from all of the participants, and found that those eating the live active yogurt had significantly higher levels of infection-battling gamma interferon (a protein crucial to a strong immune system); their interferon levels were five times higher than the group not eating yogurt.

In a second study at UC Davis, participants who ate a cup of live active yogurt a day were 25 percent less likely to develop colds than their counterparts who didn't eat yogurt. Even when the yogurt-eaters caught colds, they recovered from them faster.

If you want to put yogurt to the test, read labels carefully. Look for the statement that the yogurt contains "live and active cultures"; according to industry guidelines, that means that it has ten million or more live organisms per gram. These live active cultures are typically *streptococcus thermophilus, lactobacillus acidophilus,* or *lactobacillus bulgaricus.*

Healing from the Hive

At the first sign of a cold or sore throat, millions of people brew up some hot tea and drip a little honey into it. Perhaps this therapy began as an old wives' tale, but the scientific buzz is that the honeybee may be responsible for plenty of healing.

When you're struggling with a sore throat or the flu, medical anthropologist John Heinerman, Ph.D., advises making a beeline for propolis, a resinous substance gathered by bees from the leaf buds or bark of trees. It's available in health-food stores in capsules and tincture, and according to Dr. Heinerman, a study in Sarajevo several years ago during an influenza outbreak found that it was a flu fighter. Among students taking propolis in a nursing college, only 7 percent came down with the flu, compared to 63 percent of those who didn't use it. A Russian study of 260 people with throat inflammation reported relief in 90 percent of patients taking propolis.

On those occasions when Dr. Heinerman's own throat is inflamed with agonizing, all-consuming pain—the kind of sore throat that's so raw that you can't even swallow your own saliva—he grabs propolis in liquid form, taking it at night. "I use 60-percent-strength bee propolis from a company called Montana Naturals International," he says. Here's what he recommends: "Tilt your head back, take an eyedropperful of propolis, and stick it into your mouth all the way past your tongue. Then release the propolis into your throat. It may burn for a few moments, but then you'll be able to start swallowing again. By morning, your sore throat should be gone. It's the best thing I've found.''

Another of Dr. Heinerman's favorite natural remedies for sore throats: Stir 1 tablespoon of honey into a cup of hot water; add 1 teaspoon of bee pollen and 1 teaspoon of fresh lemon juice. Stir and then sip slowly.

CHICKEN SOUP—A.K.A. "JEWISH PENICILLIN"

In the twelfth century, the physician Moses Maimonides offered the following pronouncement: ''Soup made from an old chicken is of benefit against chronic fevers ... and also aids the cough.'' Since then, millions of grandmothers have turned to chicken soup as the ''medication'' of choice when a cold strikes. Often called ''Jewish penicillin,'' it certainly is comforting, even if there isn't anything miraculous about it.

For many years, scientists have wondered whether there was more myth than fact surrounding chicken soup. So in 1978, Marvin Sackner, M.D., of Mt. Sinai Hospital in Miami Beach studied the ability of chicken soup (obtained from a neighborhood delicatessen) to break up congestion and clear secretions from the nasal passages; he compared it with the activity of hot and cold water. Volunteers consumed all the liquids through a straw, sometimes from a covered cup and other times from an open one, and researchers measured the speed at which the mucus drained from their nasal passages. The investigators found that while cold water slowed the flow of mucus, both hot water and chicken soup accelerated the drainage, with the chicken soup beating the

hot water by a nose. Because these positive effects were
seen when the soup was in the open cup, it appeared
that the hot vapors and the aroma emanating from the
soup, when inhaled, played a role; they also stimulated
the cilia in the nose and the mucus flow more effectively
than the vapors from the hot water. However, 30 minutes
after the experiment had ended, the nasal congestion returned, indicating that the benefits of chicken soup, although soothing, were short-lived.

In a journal article describing his study, Dr. Sackner
wrote that consuming the hot fluids ''increases nasal mucus velocity because of inhalation of heated water vapor.
Hot chicken soup, either through its aroma or a mechanism related to taste, appears to possess an additional
substance which increases nasal mucus velocity.''

Then in 1993, at the University of Nebraska Medical
Center, Stephen Rennard, M.D., conducted a study using
his wife's chicken soup, prepared from a family recipe.
Dr. Rennard found that extracts of the soup stimulated
the activity of white blood cells and quieted the inflammatory response associated with symptoms such as mucus production and airway soreness. However, it did not
kill the cold virus, and thus provided only symptomatic
relief—which isn't bad, either!

''Chicken soup does work for colds,'' says infectious-
diseases specialist Steven Mostow, M.D., although the
ingredient or the mechanism that soothes cold symptoms
hasn't yet been confirmed. Nevertheless, there are a lot
of theories as to how this golden broth may work. Dr.
Rennard hypothesized that the credit belongs to perhaps
hundreds of compounds found in the vegetables used to
prepare the chicken soup. Botanist James Duke, Ph.D.,
simply says that ''hot helps''; he suggests making the

chicken soup spicy, adding plenty of hot red pepper as well as garlic and onions (which may have anti-inflammatory effects). Add to that the TLC that comes with every bowl, and you may have the answer.

So should you try chicken soup for a cold? Can't hurt!

3

Supplements: Can They Stem the Tide?

When Nobel laureate Linus Pauling was touting vitamin C as something of a miracle worker capable of wiping out the common cold, it seemed too good to be true. Maybe it was.

Without a doubt, vitamins and minerals—in our foods and in supplements—are valuable allies in the war on colds. But Dr. Pauling's pronouncements may have been overly optimistic, and not always supported by the evidence. Even so, there's still reason to think that vitamin C—not to mention other crucial vitamin supplements—can smother some of the physiological processes that lead to a sniffling nose.

Are supplements really necessary? Well, if you're counting only on your diet to supply your vitamin and mineral needs, you may have to put your food intake into overdrive. Many Americans don't even reach the RDAs (Recommended Dietary Allowances) in their meals, much less the higher amounts that may be necessary to really clobber a cold. Art Ulene, M.D., the author of *The Vitamin Strategy*, says that the optimal intake of vitamin C is 250 to 500 mg a day. But the government's 1994 statistics show that the per capita daily intake of C is only 99 mg. The same is true for vitamin E; according to Dr. Ulene, the optimal daily intake is 100 to 200 international units (IU), although the average American woman gets barely 10 IU per day. No wonder many people are filling up their shopping carts not only with food, but also with bottles of vitamin pills.

In this chapter, we'll discuss the vitamin and mineral supplements that can help you ward off the sneezes and sniffles this cold season.

THE OLD MAN AND THE C

Until his death in 1994, Linus Pauling never wavered from his stance as a true believer in vitamin C. Inspired by his vision, millions of people still are Pauling disciples, bathing themselves in vitamin C.

The RDA for vitamin C is a mere 60 mg—enough to give deficiency diseases such as scurvy the cold shoulder, but certainly not enough to send your handkerchief into premature retirement. In his book *Vitamin C and the Common Cold* Pauling recommended taking megadoses of the vitamin—1,000 to 2,000 mg a day, increasing to 4,000 to 10,000 mg when you have a cold. He believed that this regimen would produce 45 percent fewer colds, and a 60 percent decrease in the duration of these colds. Pauling suspected that vitamin C's effectiveness against colds could be "attributed to its action in strengthening the intercellular cement and in this way preventing or hindering the motion of the virus particles through the tissue and into the cells.'' Although high doses of vitamin C are generally safe (the body excretes what it doesn't need), some people have complained of adverse effects (diarrhea, abdominal cramps, headaches) associated with mega-amounts. Many experts question whether the intake really needs to be as high as Pauling advised.

Is there a happy compromise between the RDA and Pauling's prescription? Let's look at the research. There have been dozens of studies (some more scientifically sound than others), and the weight of the evidence shows that while vitamin C can reduce the severity and duration of a cold that you already have, it is less successful in actually preventing colds. Here are some of the findings:

- In 1995, investigators at the University of Helsinki evaluated the existing studies of vitamin C and the common cold, and reached encouraging conclusions: They found that high doses of vitamin C (1 to 6 grams per day—or up to 100 times the RDA!) decreased the severity of symptoms in cold sufferers by 21 percent, while reducing the length of the average cold by about one day. Their bottom line: ''Vitamin C significantly decreases the duration of episodes of the common cold.''
- Virologist Elliot Dick of the University of Wisconsin–Madison has conducted a series of similar studies beginning in the mid-1980s, all of them showing that vitamin C can reduce the severity of cold symptoms. In his research, he gave a daily dose of either 2 grams of vitamin C (in four 500-mg tablets) or a placebo (sugar pill) to 48 volunteers for three

weeks; then he assigned them to play cards for an entire weekend with people who were sneezing their way through terrible colds. While about the same number of volunteers from each group caught colds—showing that vitamin C provided no preventive benefits—those who developed colds and took vitamin C ended up putting their symptoms into cold storage more quickly—blowing their noses less frequently and coughing less often.

- There may be at least one group for whom vitamin C may have preventive powers. For long-distance runners and marathoners, a 1996 study at the University of Helsinki might be particularly good news, and encourage athletes to keep a bottle of vitamin C beside their running shoes. The Finnish researchers found that high doses of vitamin C (600 to 1,000 mg a day) reduced the number of colds in these athletes by about half.

- In 1997 at Carnegie Mellon University in Pittsburgh, Sheldon Cohen, Ph.D., and his research team evaluated lifestyle habits, including a possible association between vitamin C intake and the risk of colds. The investigators concluded that people who consumed more than 85 mg of vitamin C a day had a decreased likelihood of catching a cold than those who took it in lower amounts.

Some researchers believe that the efficacy of vitamin C is linked with its ability to increase the levels of lymphocytes, a key immune-system warrior. It also gives a boost to an antioxidant called *glutathione*, which contributes to a healthy immune system. In a study at the U.S. Department of Agriculture, a 500-mg dose of vitamin C sent levels of glutathione soaring.

What's the sum and substance of vitamin C therapy? At the first sign of a cold, increase your vitamin C consumption for several days, in hopes that it will keep your symptoms from stampeding over your body. Kenneth Cooper, M.D., the author of *Advanced Nutritional Therapies*, believes that the optimum dose of vitamin C is 2,000 to 3,000 mg a day when you feel a cold developing, or if you already have one.

Spread out your intake over the day—taking equal doses two to four times over a 24-hour period—to minimize any side effects and to keep your blood levels of vitamin C high; the body rids itself of vitamin C in about 12 hours, and thus you need to replenish it at regular intervals. If you're taking massive doses of vitamin C— for example, more than 8 grams a day—be particularly alert for the development of side effects. Avoid taking megadoses of *chewable* vitamin C tablets, which can damage the teeth by dissolving enamel.

Medical anthropologist John Heinerman, Ph.D., believes that combining plenty of vitamin C with a good mineral supplement can enhance the efficacy of vitamin C alone. In one of his studies, a group of patients took a form of vitamin C called *ester C* in a dose of 500 mg three times a day. A second group consumed the same dose of vitamin C, but also added ten to twelve drops of a liquid mineral supplement called ConcenTrace, taken in a glass of water. "The people taking the minerals plus the C had a quicker recovery from colds and flu," he says. The reason? Dr. Heinerman believes that the minerals keep vitamin C in the circulating blood plasma for longer periods of time.

Natural or Synthetic: Does It Really Matter?

If you browse through the shelves of your local pharmacy or health-food store, you'll see vitamin supplement labels proclaiming that their contents are either "natural" or "synthetic." The natural vitamins generally cost more—sometimes a lot more—and there's certainly some appeal attached to the word *natural*. But does it really make a difference?

Most objective vitamin experts say no. While the natural supplements are made from food, and the synthetic products are concocted in a chemist's beaker, your body will never be able to tell the difference. As Art Ulene, M.D., author of *The Vitamin Strategy*, says, "Despite the hype, the natural and synthetic formulations of each nutrient have the same chemical configuration, whether they were obtained from plants or made in a laboratory. Once you remove them from the bottle and swallow them, they act identically."

In vitamin E and beta-carotene, there actually are very minor differences between the natural and synthetic chemical formulations. But they are so subtle that they really don't account for any significant differences once they enter your body.

Keep in mind that there are no FDA guidelines regulating what the word *natural* really means. As a result, *natural* is defined just the way the manufacturer wants it defined. Some "natural" products may actually be a *blend* of synthetic and plant products. If you're going to buy "natural," choose a major manufacturer that you feel you can trust.

IS E FOR EVERYONE?

There is no shortage of astonishing claims about those amber-colored, almost-see-through capsules of vitamin E—that it prevents or slows coronary heart disease, certain cancers, cataracts, arthritis, diabetes, Alzheimer's disease, Parkinson's disease, and even wrinkles. Some of these claims are more hype than substance, but on balance, those vitamin E pills appear to be worth popping, including when your goal is boosting immune function and thus clobbering the common cold.

Vitamin E is really a generic term encompassing a number of compounds called *tocopherols* and *tocotrienols*. It functions as an antioxidant within the body, crippling and mopping up disease-promoting free radicals and thus minimizing and preventing the damage to healthy cell membranes. Your body needs vitamin E to operate at or near peak levels, using its extra clout to fight off cold viruses and other invading substances. Here is what some of the research shows:

- In a 1997 study led by Tufts University researchers, 88 healthy people over age 65 were evaluated for the effects of vitamin E supplementation on their immune function. Half of them took one of three daily doses of vitamin E (60, 200, or 800 IU), and the other half took a placebo. After four months, those consuming the vitamin E showed improvement in their immunological responses. The greatest increases were seen in the people taking 200 IU of vitamin E, although the investigators offered no clear-cut explanation of why those on the 200-IU regimen fared better than those taking the higher

(800-IU) dose. (Perhaps the lesson is that more is not always better.) Best of all for the anti-cold campaign, all the volunteers taking vitamin E supplements in this study had a 30 percent lower incidence of colds and flu than the placebo group.

- In another study at Tufts University in 1990, 32 healthy men and women (age 60 and over) took either a high daily dose of vitamin E (800 IU) or a placebo. After four weeks, the investigators measured a number of immune-system parameters and found upward trends in white-blood-cell response and skin-test reactions; by comparison, there were no changes in the placebo group. Those taking vitamin E actually had an immune function comparable to that of much younger individuals.
- In yet another study, Czech scientists gave nursing-home residents a daily dose of 450 IU of vitamin E and 1,000 mg of vitamin C. Compared to a control group, these individuals had fewer viral infections and a lower mortality rate from the flu.
- In an animal study at Tufts University, older mice were fed either very high doses of vitamin E or much more modest amounts of the vitamin (6 percent of the levels given to the first group). Then, after two months, all of the mice were exposed to the flu virus. Researchers found that the mice that had received the megadoses seemed much better prepared for a fight; they had much lower levels of the virus in their lungs than those getting the reduced doses of vitamin E. Interestingly, however, when *younger* mice were given vitamin E, huge amounts offered no more protection than the lower dose. Based on these findings, the researchers hy-

pothesized that in humans, vitamin E's benefits in preventing the flu may be most helpful in older individuals.

How much vitamin E do you need? If you believe the RDAs, all your body requires is 15 IU (for men) or 12 IU (for women) a day. But studies suggest that most Americans aren't even getting those levels (70 percent of adult women don't reach the RDA through their diets alone), let alone the much higher amounts of vitamin E that they *really* require to enjoy all of its benefits, including its possible help in overwhelming cold viruses. Remember, despite what the RDAs say, the *optimal* dose of vitamin E may be at least 100 IU (some researchers believe it's much higher). So even though you can find vitamin E in a number of foods, it's virtually impossible to get as much as you need through diet alone, particularly if you're eating low-fat foods. Just consider these numbers: To reach 100 IU, you'd have to eat 5 cups of wild rice, 3 glasses of whole milk, 5 tablespoons of safflower oil, *and* 20 dried prunes. It would be even more challenging to reach higher intake levels of 200 to 800 IU.

The good news is that even at high supplemental doses of vitamin E, there's usually no worry about side effects; studies show that for most people, high doses of vitamin E are safe. However, if you take anticoagulant drugs or have a deficiency in vitamin K, talk to your doctor before self-prescribing vitamin E.

THINK ZINC!

Is there magic in minerals? It may seem that way, at least where zinc is concerned.

Some researchers, it seems, can't stop talking about zinc. They believe that no mineral is more important to a strong immune system. They'll tell you that when you're not getting enough of it, your immunity may pay the price. As your zinc intake falls, so might your levels of infection-busting white blood cells. But by boosting your zinc consumption, you might breathe new life into your body's infection-fighting potential, and give colds a very cool reception.

Investigators at the University of Medicine and Dentistry in New Jersey (UMDNJ) have found that just a modest amount of zinc each day—15 mg, which is the RDA for male adults—invigorates the immune system, especially in people over age 50. That might help ambush the sniffles before they even start. In a study in Italy, when a 15-mg daily dose of zinc was given to people over age 65, their T-cell levels soared as high as those seen in much younger adults.

Keep track of your intake of zinc, however. If you down it by the handful, you could be courting disaster. "When zinc is consumed in high doses or even in moderate amounts over a long period, it can actually *depress* your immune function," says John Bogden, Ph.D., professor of preventive medicine and community health at UMDNJ. To complicate matters, he adds, some research shows that high doses of zinc may *decrease* HDL cholesterol—the "good" cholesterol that you'd like to keep at dizzying heights.

So what's the optimal dose of zinc? Ranjit Chandra, M.D., a pediatrician and immune-function researcher at Memorial University of Newfoundland, believes that 25 mg of zinc a day is best—about 10 mg from your diet, and another 15 mg from supplements. (See the adjoining box for good sources of dietary zinc.)

Think Zinc! Where to Find It

The best sources of zinc in the diet are red meat, wheat germ, and oysters. But many foods provide this important mineral, including the following:

beef	turkey	chicken
corned beef	vegetable soup	kidney beans
flank steak	yogurt	lentils
wheat germ	ricotta cheese	lima beans
miso	black beans	pinto beans
oysters	cashews	navy beans
crab	black-eyed peas	lobster
liver	carrots	Manhattan
		clam chowder

Besides zinc tablets and zinc-rich foods, there's another form in which zinc can protect you from the cold bug—namely, zinc lozenges. In recent times, zinc lozenges have become something of a medical fad, gaining enormous popularity after a highly publicized study at the Cleveland Clinic was published in the *Annals of Internal Medicine* in 1996. The genesis of this brouhaha over lozenges dates back to the early 1980s, when a man from Texas made a serendipitous discovery. His 3-year-old daughter was being treated for leukemia with chemotherapy, and one night she fell asleep while sucking on a zinc lozenge, one of a number of supplements prescribed to keep her as nutritionally sound as possible. She had been suffering from a cold, but recovered from it more quickly than usual this time. Although not a scientist, the father began researching the therapeutic benefits of zinc; his work eventually snowballed into a flurry of studies on zinc lozenges.

Then came the Cleveland Clinic study. Researchers there gave zinc lozenges (called Cold-Eeze) to men and women who had developed cold symptoms within the previous 24 hours; another group of patients with colds received placebos. The lozenges were taken every two hours while the subjects were awake—with startling results. Most of the cold symptoms (runny nose, nasal congestion, sore throat, headache, hoarseness, coughs) of the zinc users lasted a much shorter time (an average of three days less than the placebo group)—persisting an average of 4.4 days, compared to 7.6 days for those getting the placebo; this means that those receiving zinc recovered almost twice as fast as the placebo poppers. However, there was no difference between the two groups in the resolution of several other symptoms (fever, sneezing, muscle aches).

In the Cleveland Clinic research, the lozenges contained zinc gluconate (13.3 mg per lozenge); since some people consumed as many as eight lozenges per day, that's a total daily zinc intake of 106 mg—far above the RDA; nevertheless, because this regimen was followed for only a few days while cold symptoms were flaring, researchers did not consider it a reason to panic. Even so, an editorial that accompanied publication of the zinc study warned, "Surveillance for potential toxicity will be needed for a good many years if zinc therapy becomes widely adopted for one of mankind's most common and seemingly most intractable maladies.''

Were any side effects noted? Even though 80 percent of the lozenge-takers complained of an unpleasant taste (and 20 percent experienced nausea), this may have been an acceptable trade-off for hammering the cold virus into submission. The commercially available over-the-counter lozenges have citrus flavoring added to them, which has made them much more palatable, although you still won't mistake them for cherry Life Savers.

As the research continues, many cold experts are still taking a wait-and-see attitude toward zinc lozenges (to date, about half of the studies have come down on the side of zinc as a cold cure, although their benefits in children are questionable). In the meantime, scientists are hypothesizing how zinc might put a cold to rest. Although no one knows for sure, one theory is that zinc stimulates the proliferation of interferon, which is a natural infection fighter. Zinc might also interfere with the ability of the cold virus to invade cells in the lining of the respiratory tract.

If you decide to try zinc lozenges, begin popping them when you first feel a cold creeping up. Take one every two to four hours for as long as your symptoms persist.

DOES SELENIUM MAKE SENSE?

When it comes to antioxidants, selenium is like a neglected stepchild pleading for attention. It doesn't get much of the limelight, although it still goes about doing its work quietly, winning the plaudits of some scientists and making inroads into a field dominated by the anti-oxidant superstars—vitamins C and E.

Of course, it's hard to ignore the occasional study that should elevate selenium into the winner's circle—such as the Christmas Day headline in 1996 humbly proclaiming, "Selenium Prevents Cancer." That particular story, based on a study in the *Journal of the American Medical Association,* grew out of a ten-year tracking of 1,300 people. Researchers found that 200 micrograms (mcg) of selenium sharply reduced the risk of three types of cancer—lung, colon, and prostate—by 45 to 63 percent; overall, there were 50 percent fewer cancer deaths among selenium takers. Not bad for a mineral that most people still haven't heard of.

How does a trace mineral like selenium take the steam out of a life-threatening disease like cancer? Apparently by bolstering the immune system. That immune system surge is also good news when your goals are simpler than thwarting cancer—like stamping out the sniffles. In one experiment in which volunteers were given selenium intravenously (ouch!) at a dose of 200 mcg a day for two months, their immune function improved. That could be disastrous for viruses trying to scale the walls of a weakened immune system, since a strong immune function may keep them from replicating and running rampant in your respiratory tract.

Several studies in the 1990s have looked at the ability of selenium to steamroll over a type of virus called *Coxsackie virus.* It is responsible for a common infection in young children that triggers a sore throat, fever, dehydration, mouth sores, and a skin rash. Researchers have found that in people with deficiencies in selenium and vitamin E, mutations and rapid replication of the Cox-sackie virus are much more likely.

So stocking up on selenium makes sense as an insurance policy against the common cold and other illnesses. After all, there is even evidence (although not yet conclusive) that selenium may protect against heart disease. You can meet most of your selenium needs in your diet (see the adjoining box), but its levels in foods such as whole grains can vary, depending on the mineral content of the soil in which they've been grown and the water that nourished them (selenium levels tend to be lower on the coasts than in the heartland of the United States). For that reason, selenium is gradually emerging as a permanent fixture on the mineral supplement best-seller list.

The RDA for selenium is 70 mcg for men and 55 mcg for women, but you can confidently go higher than that when taking supplements. Daily doses of 100 to 200 mcg are safe and appear capable of toughening up the immune system. However, don't climb beyond 200 mcg of supplementation; if you exceed that level, you might be tempting toxicity (although reports of serious side effects are uncommon). Levels greater than 700 mcg have been associated with tooth loss, nerve damage, diarrhea, fatigue, fragile fingernails, hair loss, and garlic-like bad breath.

Selenium Sources

Where should you steer your shopping cart when looking for selenium-rich foods? Here are some good places to start:

haddock	walnuts	spinach
crab	brazil nuts	green peas
pork chops	chicken	mushrooms
salmon	apricots	onions
kidney beans	grapefruit	oranges
beef liver	carrots	turnips
leg of lamb	celery	ham
turkey breast	low-fat yogurt	sunflower seeds
oysters	egg yolks	
cashews	avocados	

MAKE ROOM FOR MULTIVITAMINS

Long before their pantry shelves were lined with rows of vitamin bottles, many people relied on a single multivitamin-and-mineral supplement to help them reach nutritional nirvana. Some still do.

Of course, there's nothing particularly trendy, nor anything to create much of a buzz, about these unpretentious one-a-day pills. But if your goal is combating colds and keeping your immune system strong as it goes into battle, then that single, simple pill should take its rightful place at or near the front lines.

In 1994, a study published in the *American Journal of Clinical Nutrition* by Ranjit Chandra, M.D., and his colleagues at Memorial University of Newfoundland, concluded that when a daily multivitamin supplement was used by older people over the long term, it enhanced the strength of their immune systems. Remember, immune function tends to decline with age in some individuals, but a multivitamin-and-mineral pill may be able to plug up the leaks and compensate for deficiencies. In this particular study, 56 healthy people (age 59 and over) were given either a Theragran-M multivitamin tablet or a placebo each day for a year. The multivitamin contained most nutrients in levels comparable to the RDAs, but with higher amounts of vitamin E and beta-carotene. After a year, the researchers measured the nutrient blood levels of the volunteers and also conducted skin tests, which consist of injecting foreign substances that could cause infections or diseases and monitoring how the immune system responds to them.

The results? Researchers found higher concentrations of the supplemented nutrients in the bloodstreams of the multivitamin group, including significantly increased levels of vitamins C and E, folic acid, and beta-carotene. At the same time, their immune-system responses increased 64 percent and they had higher amounts of natural killer cells, which can fight off viruses and cancerous cells. Clearly, their immune function was better equipped to flatten infections than it had been when the study began. In short, the study provided a resounding vote of confidence for multivitamin-and-mineral supplements.

In an earlier study in *The Lancet* by the same researchers, 96 healthy men and women over age 65 took a supplement containing eighteen vitamins and minerals. Over the course of a year, the pill users had significantly fewer infections than the non-users, and were ill with infections for only half the number of days—an average of 23 days, compared with 48 days in the placebo group. The most common of these sicknesses were colds, flus, bronchitis, and sinus infections. Blood measurements showed increases in levels of zinc, iron, beta-carotene, and vitamins A, B$_6$, and C in the supplement takers, and improvements in immune-system parameters such as T-cells, lymphocyte responses, and natural killer cells.

Keep in mind, advises John Bogden, Ph.D., that "even mild deficiencies of some micronutrients can compromise immunity." But he also cautions that you can't expect instant results from a multivitamin-and-mineral supplement. "Low-dose multivitamins require six months or more to improve immunity, although they may do so sooner in men than in women," he says.

So what should you choose if you want to try this "one-for-all and all-in-one" approach? There are dozens of multivitamin-and-mineral supplements on the market. Some can be swallowed; others are chewed. Some contain more nutrients than others. But no matter which brand you select, you've chosen a simple way to tackle deficiencies in your immune function and improve the odds of slaying the common-cold dragon before it starts breathing fire.

4

Healing with Herbs

Let's start with a definition: An herb is a plant that can be used for medicinal purposes. Herbs are used to treat and protect against illnesses, and have played these roles for millennia. You'll find them available as pills or in their natural plant form for chopping or squeezing into other dishes during cooking, or for brewing in a tea.

Herbs are particularly popular in Asia, where they are essential components of the health-care system. In Europe, they are carefully regulated by a multi-tiered network established by the European Community, which provides standards that must be followed by manufacturers. In the United States, however, many people still eye them skeptically.

But before you instinctively recoil at the thought of using herbs, wondering how you could possibly rely on a plant to prevent or treat colds or more serious illnesses, consider this fact: Many of Western medicine's most popular and reliable drugs—about 25 percent of them, in fact—have had their origin in plants. Salicin, the foundation of everyday aspirin, comes from willow tree bark; digitalis, the heart drug, is derived from the foxglove plant; and taxol, the cancer chemotherapeutic agent, comes from the Pacific yew tree.

That isn't all. You probably also rely on an herb (coffee) to perk you up in the morning. You might turn to another herb (aloe vera) to keep your skin moist. In many cases, the precise mechanism of even the most popular herbs is not well understood, but that's not surprising: There's not a complete understanding of how many mainstream pharmaceuticals work, either.

Unless you count health-food stores among your favorite haunts, you may not have even heard of some of the herbs we'll discuss in this chapter. But the evidence suggests that herbs can often leave you breathing easier when you're assaulted by a cold, with a more natural and less costly road to recovery than the manufactured medications that come out of pharmaceutical labs.

Buyer Beware: Does It Apply to Herbs?

A survey by *Prevention* magazine in 1997 found that one-third of adults in the United States spend an average of $54 a year on herbal supplements. But although herbal remedies have a growing army of proponents, many experts urge consumer caution in selecting these supplements. That's because herbal products are considered dietary supplements, not drugs, and thus they aren't regulated by the Food and Drug Administration in the way that the agency oversees medications (both prescription and nonprescription). A relatively new government agency, the Office of Dietary Supplements Research, monitors nutritional supplements and the claims made by manufacturers; however, it doesn't enforce the same strict regulations as the FDA, which requires elaborate premarketing evaluation for effectiveness and safety before a drug is approved for sale.

Of course, you might think you have something important on your side—namely, that herbal remedies are derived from plants. Even so, they can't be taken in unlimited amounts (depending on the herb, toxicity symptoms could include a rash, diarrhea, and/or stomach upset). To protect yourself, find out as much as you can about a particular herb before you try it. Buy from a manufacturer whose name you recognize, and look for the term *standardized* on the label; this indicates that the company ensures that the strength and potency of its products are uniform in every pill. Don't exceed the recommended dose on the label. Better yet, follow the guidelines of an experienced practitioner of herbal medicine.

ECHINACEA

Most people can't pronounce *echinacea*, (its most common pronunciation is *eck-in-NAY-sha*), much less tell you what it is. Also called *purple coneflower*, it's a member of the daisy family; before it became popular among cold sufferers, it had been used for centuries in this country for wound healing (it was commonly applied to snakebites by Native Americans).

The theory behind echinacea is that it increases the number and stimulates the activity of leukocytes (white blood cells), and sends them in for the kill, devouring cold and flu viruses. It may also accelerate the body's production of interferon, a natural virus-fighter that prevents viral replication and triggers a process that destroys viruses. Botanist James Duke, Ph.D., the author of *The Green Pharmacy,* says that the herb contains several chemicals—chicoric acid, caffeic acid, and echinacin—that can catch viruses in their crosshairs. "Echinacea won't dry up the membranes in your nasal passages," says Theodore Robertson, M.D., who practices mind-body wellness in Coronado, California. "But it provides cellular-mediated immune stimulation."

There have been hundreds of studies of echinacea, but most don't meet the scientific rigors that doctors prefer to see (that's also the case with the majority of other herbs, since there isn't much incentive for companies to fund carefully controlled studies of plants that can't be patented anyway!). Nevertheless, the German Institute for Drugs and Medical Devices (Germany's counterpart to our FDA) has moved echinacea to the head of the class, approving it for treating colds and flus.

Here is what some of the best research on echinacea has shown:

- In a German study in 1992, nearly 200 people with the flu (ages 18 to 60) were given high doses of *Echinacea purpurea* extract. Those taking 180 drops (800 mg), the equivalent of four droppersful of echinacea, experienced a 75 percent decline in their flu symptoms (sore throat, muscle pains, stuffy nose, fatigue) in three to four days; this dose was twice as effective as a placebo. But those taking a lower dose—90 drops a day—fared no better than the placebo group.

- In another 1992 German study, researchers gave echinacea to 108 cold-prone people (ages 13 to 84) as part of a juice mixture; these individuals had experienced three or more bouts of the sniffles during the previous winter. The volunteers took 4 milliliters of *Echinacea purpurea,* twice a day, for eight weeks. The herb reduced their risk of catching a cold by 36 percent, compared to a placebo group, while also minimizing the severity and duration of the colds they did develop.
- In 1994, a comprehensive review of 26 studies of echinacea by German researchers found that the herb could fight infections (colds, flus) and stimulate the activity of the immune system.

Echinacea is available as liquid extracts, capsules, tablets, and teas. Look for standardized formulations and for particular preparations. Though there are nine species of echinacea, only two have been studied extensively; choose products derived from *Echinacea purpurea* or *Echinacea angustifolia.*

"I recommend echinacea to my patients for colds," says George A. Ulett, M.D., Ph.D., clinical professor in the Department of Community and Family Medicine at the St. Louis University School of Medicine. "I advise using the fluid extract of echinacea. Put 15 drops in one-quarter of a glass of water, and swish it around in your mouth before you swallow it. That's because you want to boost the immune system in your throat and respiratory system in particular." Dr. Ulett, the author of *Al-*

ternative Medicine or Magical Healing, suggests taking echinacea (along with 1,000 mg of vitamin C and a zinc lozenge under the tongue) three times a day for five days when you're coping with a cold. Then put the herb back on the shelf, and don't use it again until the next time you're exposed to a cold or when your nose starts to run. "If you immediately go to echinacea, you'll find symptoms disappearing in 24 to 48 hours," he says.

There's some evidence that your body will build up a tolerance to echinacea, and thus its efficacy could wane if used all the time. For that reason, German doctors have recommended that echinacea not be taken for longer than eight-week stretches. In the United States, botanist James Duke, Ph.D., is a leading proponent of letting echinacea stay on the shelf except when it's needed; but when the flu bug is running rampant in his community, or when he's in contact with people who have colds, Dr. Duke will fill up on echinacea capsules.

By the way, if you decide to try the liquid extract of echinacea, brace yourself for a taste that might send you lunging for some mouthwash. The flavor of echinacea has been compared to that of tree bark (which isn't much of a delicacy). Some people can't get used to it, and settle for the capsules instead.

Recommended dosages can vary, so carefully read the labels of the product you buy.

Caution: Who Shouldn't Take Echinacea?

Not everyone should reach for echinacea when a cold or the flu strikes. Because of the herb's unique influence on the immune system, you should avoid it if you have rheumatoid arthritis, lupus, multiple sclerosis, or type I diabetes. Also stay away from echinacea if you're allergic to plants in the daisy family (to which echinacea belongs).

The side effects associated with echinacea are mild or nonexistent. Diarrhea and an upset stomach are the most commonly reported adverse effects. Nevertheless, herbal practitioners generally recommend that children and pregnant women give the cold shoulder to *all* herbs—including echinacea—unless they're under the care and guidance of a physician.

GOLDENSEAL

It may sound like the name of a marine animal that you're more likely to encounter at Sea World than at a health-food store. But goldenseal is all the buzz in the world of herbs, and consistently ranks among the top five herbal best-sellers. When it comes to the common cold, if echinacea doesn't completely plug up your nasal drip, goldenseal might put the final seal on it. At least that's the hope.

Goldenseal is a perennial forest plant—botanists call it *Hydrastis canadensis*—and it grows particularly well in moist, shady areas. But because *Hydrastis canadenis* is a real tongue-twister, its more popular name, drawn from its sharp golden coloring, has caught on. Although goldenseal's early uses by Native Americans (especially the Cherokee) included caring for minor skin conditions and rinsing out irritated eyes, scientific attention has now turned toward the herb's ability to boost the immune system by stimulating infection-fighting white blood cells. When you're seeking a way to mug the cold bug, some herb experts advise getting more bang for the buck by combining echinacea with goldenseal. The hope is that when you strengthen your immune function, cold symptoms will wave the white flag.

As with many herbs, however, formal research into goldenseal has been scarce. Botanist James Duke, Ph.D., believes that berberine, one of goldenseal's active ingredients, stimulates the activity of macrophages, which in turn leaves viruses and bacteria screaming for mercy. He carries goldenseal and echinacea with him in his travel remedy kit. Skeptics, however, have pointed out that when consumed, the active components of goldenseal (including berberine and hydrastine) may have to fight their way into the bloodstream; if they don't make it all the way there, the herb might not have much influence on immune function. Goldenseal may work better as a topical antiseptic for sore throats, and that seems to be one reason people are grabbing it off the shelf. Goldenseal acts like a mild anesthetic when it makes contact with tissues in the throat; if it hurts to swallow, gargling with a potion of goldenseal might be worth a try. Varro Tyler, Ph.D., Sc.D., a herbal expert at Purdue University, says that goldenseal tea is often used as a rinse to ease cracked lips and canker sores.

Until 1936, goldenseal was actually included in the *U.S. Pharmacopoeia*, where it was listed as an antiseptic; but it fell out of favor when antibiotics began taking center stage. In even earlier times, it was a prominent ingredient in many nineteenth-century patent medicines (one of them carried the rather modest name of "Dr. Pierce's Golden Medical Discovery"). More recently, goldenseal has gathered a growing following in the United States for quite another reason: Back in the 1970s, when drug testing was entering mainstream America, myths arose that by popping a little goldenseal, you could camouflage your use of everything from marijuana to heroin. Thousands of people, from corporate employees to athletes, began taking goldenseal as an "antidote" to illicit drugs that might show up in a urine test. But in fact, there has never been any scientific evidence to support goldenseal's ability to either flush drugs from the system or prevent their detection. Herb experts have traced these inaccurate claims to a researcher who had made them in a novel—not a scientific journal—that he wrote around the turn of the century. But undeterred by the notion that goldenseal's support came in a work of fiction, people concerned about passing a drug test began popping goldenseal as though it were candy.

Should you try goldenseal to treat a cold? Its greatest efficacy may rest with its ability to spell relief for a sore throat. So when you're suffering with a sore throat, head to the health-food store. Follow the label instructions for dosage; in a typical formulation, you might mix ½ teaspoon of goldenseal powder (or the contents of a goldenseal capsule) into a cup of hot water, and gargle with it four or more times a day; use honey to counteract its generally bitter flavor.

One important caveat: There is some evidence that

when taken internally, goldenseal might increase blood pressure in some people, so talk to your doctor if you already have hypertension. Pregnant women should avoid goldenseal as well, because of concerns that it might trigger uterine contractions.

ASTRAGALUS

In Chinese medicine, an herb called astragalus is considered an excellent infection fighter, and is the best herbal immunity booster. Not only is it used to fight colds and flus, but it is recommended for more serious illnesses, too. Also known as *huang qi* or milk vetch, astragalus is the root of a plant (*Astragalus membranaceous*) in the pea family.

In China, astragalus is sold in drugstores as a cold fighter with the same enthusiasm with which Sudafed and Contac are promoted here. It is sometimes recommended for patients undergoing cancer chemotherapy to strengthen immune systems weakened by potent treatments. But its antiviral properties have won the most attention.

As with many herbs, astragalus and its use are supported more by anecdotal reports than by carefully controlled scientific studies. Limited research in the United States and particularly in China, however, suggest that astragalus may be able to increase the activity of the immune system, including interferon (a virus-fighting substance) and natural killer cells, and improve resistance to colds and other infections. At M.D. Anderson Cancer Center at the University of Texas, investigators conducted tests in the laboratory to evaluate the effects of chemicals in astragalus upon cells taken from patients with cancer and other life-threatening viral diseases (including AIDS). They found that astragalus increased the activity and responsiveness of natural defenses such as disease-fighting T-cells.

Most health-food stores sell astragalus as either capsules or tinctures. A capsule or two a day is a typical dosage unless you have a chronic respiratory illness such as bronchitis or sinusitis, but again, be sure to read dosage guidelines on the label of the specific item you choose. Some products combine half a dozen or more Chinese herbs, including astragalus, in a single capsule. In shops that sell Chinese herbs, or from Chinese practitioners themselves, you can also obtain dried astragalus root and use slices of it in preparing tea or soup.

Astragalus has a good safety profile. Nevertheless, there have been reports of minor side effects such as diarrhea and abdominal pain in some patients.

LICORICE

If you bought candy like Good & Plenty at the movie theater when you were a kid, you might have been doing more than satisfying your sweet tooth. The licorice in the candy may have kept you cough-free for the duration of the movie, thanks to an active chemical called glycyrrhizin.

Of course, this is the news that children (and most adults) have been waiting for: Eating candy is good for your health! In fact, licorice is an herb that, according to recent research, really can help calm a cough, soothe a sore throat—and more. That doesn't surprise herbal practitioners in China and other countries, where licorice has been used for centuries to heal respiratory illnesses.

In Japan, licorice extract is also used as a treatment for the viral disease hepatitis B and for bacterial diseases (*Streptococci* and *Staphylococci* infections). It may stimulate the release of the antiviral compound interferon within the body and block viral replication. Years ago, Dutch researchers claimed that licorice also could help heal peptic ulcers.

Andrew Weil, M.D., of the University of Arizona's Program in Integrative Medicine, believes that licorice could have some anti-inflammatory properties; thus, it might be helpful not only for an irritated throat, but also as an adjunct to traditional arthritis medication (with your doctor's supervision). Some animal research in Japan even suggests that by strengthening the immune system, glycyrrhizin might help prevent certain cancers, particularly breast and colon cancer, although this research is quite preliminary.

For years, licorice has also been winning converts among those who prefer something more natural than a cough medication sold in the neighborhood pharmacy. Licorice seems capable of coating and soothing the mucous membranes in the respiratory tract, thus reducing irritation and coughing.

Licorice (*Glycyrrhiza glabra*) is a tall plant that grows in warm climates. For medicinal purposes, herbal practitioners sometimes combine it with herbs such as goldenseal, not only to provide an extra infection-fighting boost but also to add sweet flavoring to the mix (glycyrrhizin is 50 times sweeter than simple table sugar!). One of the most popular formulations of licorice is a lozenge combining both licorice and menthol (sold under brand names such as Lakerol). Keep in mind, however, that you need to read labels carefully when buying licorice. Some products don't contain licorice at all, but rather licorice taste-alikes (such as anise oil, which is part of the parsley family). Only the real thing can corral your cough, so avoid candies that contain ''licorice flavor'' but no glycyrrhizin.

In health-food stores, when you're shopping for licorice, you can find more than lozenges. Licorice root comes in powder form, which can be brewed in a tea; generally, just a pinch of licorice in a cup of hot herbal tea might cool a burning throat. While soothing the mucous membranes in the throat, licorice can also increase saliva flow, which is another way it quiets a cough. Buy a product from a reputable food manufacturer to ensure that you're getting good quality.

Can licorce have side effects? You bet. Some people experience minor problems such as an upset stomach or diarrhea; if that happens, stop consuming licorice, and you'll be back to normal in no time. More worrisome, however, is licorice's ability to mimic a natural hormone called aldosterone. This hormone normally regulates metabolism and keeps sodium and water in balance; but if you gorge yourself on licorice, it's like flooding your system with too much hormone, and you'll disrupt that finely tuned balance. As that happens, you might become susceptible to salt retention and potassium depletion, which could in turn raise your blood pressure, cause heart arrhythmias, or trigger headaches. Talk to your doctor about whether you're prone to conditions like these. Large amounts of licorice can also cause headaches in some people.

In his book *The Honest Herbal*, Varro Tyler, Ph.D., relates the story of a man who consumed two to three 36-gram licorice candy bars daily for six to seven years;

he became so weak that he was hospitalized for a month before regaining his strength. In another case, an elderly man chewed eight to twelve 3-ounce bags of licorice-containing chewing tobacco each day, and consistently swallowed the saliva he produced while chewing; he soon became so weak that he could no longer even sit up or raise his arms. After a period of hospitalization—during which he used no chewing tobacco—his physical health returned to normal.

Again, for the most part, these side effects occur with the consumption of large amounts of licorice extract—but they're real. Isadore Rosenfeld, M.D., the author of *Dr. Rosenfeld's Guide to Alternative Medicine*, says that "licorice-induced hypertension" is well-documented, and he advises looking for less risky ways to bring colds into submission. That's particularly good advice if you already have high blood pressure or other cardiovascular problems.

A GRAB BAG OF OTHER HERBS

Once you become sold on the possibilities of these herbs, several others may also be worth your attention while you're looking for respiratory relief. For example:

Slippery Elm

That's right, slippery elm. It's a name that hardly attracts the instant respect of someone looking for a powerful anti-cold remedy. But don't rush to judgment quite yet.

Substances obtained from the bark of the slippery elm tree were once much more prevalent and popular than they are today. Native Americans used them as a salve to treat chapped lips and burns; during the American

Revolution, surgeons treated gunshot wounds with them. Today, some health-food stores sell slippery elm–containing lozenges to soothe a sore throat, although they're not as universally available as they once were; you might need to do some Sherlock Holmes–like detective work to find them.

The magical qualities of slippery elm rest with a gummy substance or mucilage that can coat the mucous membranes in the throat and put a damper on the coughing reflex while soothing a sore throat. If you want to try it, track down some slippery elm lozenges, or place a little slippery elm powder into some hot water for a unique cup of tea. In general, the risks associated with slippery elm are limited to occasional allergic reactions. Keep your doctor informed of any possible adverse effects.

Eucalyptus

For destroying symptoms of upper respiratory infections, eucalyptus may be worth a try. By breathing in eucalyptus vapors, you might cut a cough short while easing your congestion. ''It's a good way to loosen phlegm,'' says botanist James Duke, Ph.D., noting that eucalyptus acts like an expectorant, making it easier to cough the phlegm up.

The use of eucalyptus dates back to the Australian aborigines, who relied on it to ease coughs and other virus-induced conditions. Hundreds of species of eucalyptus tree grow rampantly and large (up to 300 feet in height) in Australia; more recently, it has had a presence in North America. Although it is sometimes referred to as the Australian fever tree, there is only anecdotal evidence that it can arrest a high temperature; hundreds of years ago, eucalyptus was sometimes used for treating malaria as well, although its actual value in that area was never proven.

Where can you find eucalyptus? You may have inhaled it without giving it much thought when you've used products such as Vicks VapoRub. In some health-food stores, you can buy dried eucalyptus leaves; when they're crushed and placed in boiling water, you can brew a soothing tea in just a few minutes. Breathe in the vapors between sips, and you may get a double dose of therapy. One to two cups a day may be helpful.

Here's another alternative: Place several drops of eucalyptus oil in a warm bath and soak for a while, inhaling the fumes while you relax. Don't consume the eucalyptus oil by mouth, however; it could be poisonous if used internally.

Ginger

Growing to a height of two to four feet, the ginger plant has swordlike leaves that give it a rather ominous appearance. But don't be fooled. Pay closer attention to its aromatic flowers, and you'll get a sense of its medicinal properties.

When it comes to healing, ginger is best known for preventing motion sickness and nausea; according to Dr. Duke, ginger root was chewed by sailors thousands of years ago. But it may also help relieve colds, coughs, abdominal discomfort and, according to some proponents, even lung problems. Ginger appears to contain compounds (such as sesquiterpenes) that can combat cold viruses. Animal studies suggest that ginger may knock a few degrees off a raging fever, but no human studies have evaluated it.

You can purchase ginger as powder or in teas; ginger capsules usually contain 500 mg of the powdered herb. Use ginger in a gargle (along with a little lemon juice and honey), or sprinkle some on your dinner as a spice. You can even sip ginger ale, as long as it is made with real ginger.

Peppermint

When grandmothers aren't brewing up a bowl of steaming chicken soup to clobber the common cold, they might be preparing a cup of peppermint tea. Or they may be coaxing family members to use a peppermint gargle for sore throats, or to apply rubbing menthol (a potent constituent in peppermint) on flu-related aching muscles.

Although once confined primarily to Europe, peppermint now grows prolifically in the United States. Best known as a flavoring substance and a means for easing indigestion, peppermint appears capable of easing nasal congestion, but some proponents claim it has fever-reducing properties as well.

Most supermarkets sell pure peppermint-leaf tea. Andrew Weil, M.D., advises brewing it in a covered container to keep the volatile chemicals from being lost.

5

Stress and Your Cold

Your boss is putting the squeeze on you at work, demanding that you take on a greater workload. At home, you and your spouse argue constantly about how to balance the checkbook, and your teenager hasn't turned in a homework assignment in a month. In the midst of all of this, the freeway traffic on the way to the office has become worse than ever, and your mother has just been diagnosed with a serious illness. As your stress levels rise . . . and rise . . . and rise . . . you notice that you simply don't feel well, and your nose is starting to run.

"People who are emotionally stressed have a worse time with common cold viruses than those who handle stress well," says infectious-diseases specialist Steven Mostow, M.D. The reason? The wear and tear of constant stress appears to undermine the functioning of your immune system and your ability to fight off infections.

Of course, stress can come from a number of directions. Physical stress can be caused by a lack of sleep or by surgery. Emotional stress can arise from dozens of life circumstances, from a divorce to the death of a loved one, from a family illness to in-law troubles, from job pressures to an ominous stack of bills. As anxiety levels soar, the immune system can melt down. Lymphocyte activity plummets. Natural killer cell levels head south. In the process, you may become more susceptible to both mild and serious illnesses.

Actually, the stressful events themselves aren't what make you sick. It's the way you react to them. "The effect of stress has less to do with what's causing it, and more to do with how well you tolerate it," says David E. Bresler, Ph.D., a stress and pain specialist at the UCLA School of Medicine. "Some people fall apart in the presence of the smallest stress, but others do just fine even when confronted with severe stress."

If you take the stressful situations in your life to heart, you'll react with the so-called "fight-or-flight" response that puts the body into overdrive, and prepares it to meet the "enemy." In prehistoric times, when the caveman was confronted with a genuine threat—perhaps a tiger preparing to pounce—the body had all the physiological tools it needed to respond to the life-threatening situation. A surge of stress hormones (adrenaline, cortisol, norepinephrine) was released to instantly prepare the body to either fight or flee. The central nervous system triggered a series of biochemical reactions designed to prepare the body to defend itself. The pulse sped up. The respiration rate quickened. Blood pressure increased. Blood sugar levels climbed. Muscles tensed. Pupils became dilated. The throat tightened. He was fully prepared to respond to imminent danger.

Of course, the threats of today are quite different from

those of thousands of years ago. Saber-toothed tigers aren't roaming through most metropolitan areas, and true life-and-death situations are more the exception than the rule. They've been replaced by other menaces (deadlines at work, the fear of crime, refereeing family quarrels, paying the kids' college tuition). Although these everyday circumstances don't pose an imminent threat to our well-being, our bodies react just as they've done for centuries. As Dr. Bresler says, evolution simply hasn't kept up with the times. "We're stuck in an 'obsolete' body that, while equipped to cope with acute stress, can't adopt to the chronic anxieties of modern life," he says. Whether the threat is real or imagined, your body reacts the same way—your blood pressure climbs, your heart rate accelerates, your face becomes flushed, your muscles tense, and your stomach churns as the body shifts into a fight-or-flight response.

Once the "threat" is gone—that is, once the clogged freeway traffic begins to flow again—your body will return to its normal state. But when these stressful events repeat themselves, perhaps dozens of times during the day, chronic stress can exact a devastating toll. The average person is confronted by a staggering 20 to 40 episodes of short-term stress every day, and these frustrations can leave him or her exhausted and depressed, plagued by headaches, and bothered by upset stomachs. And as stress becomes an ugly and constant fact of life, it can sabotage the immune system. White blood cells won't react to invading organisms as aggressively as they once did. There will be declines in levels of antibodies called secretory immunoglobulin A (IgA), which stake out a position in the mucosa and create a defensive barrier against cold and flu viruses.

As stress pounds and punishes the body, the immune system may buckle, becoming more vulnerable to all kinds of illnesses—the common cold or perhaps much more serious illnesses such as asthma, heart disease, skin conditions, and perhaps even cancer.

WHAT THE RESEARCH SHOWS

The following studies have found a relationship between stress and susceptibility to colds:

- In research at Carnegie Mellon University in Pittsburgh in 1991, investigators studied about 400 healthy men and women and evaluated their stress levels by having them answer questionnaires. Then the researchers sprayed rhinovirus into the participants' noses and monitored them for the development of colds. The conclusion: The higher the stress levels, the greater the likelihood of being stricken by the sniffles. Those people with the most stress in their lives were nearly twice as likely to end up sneezing as those with the least stress.
- At Ohio State University in 1991, investigators conducted a study of 69 people who were the primary caretaker of a spouse with dementia; another 69 individuals who did not bear such responsibilities were used as a control group. After 13 months, the caretakers showed significant declines in three measurements of their immune function, compared to the controls. They also were sick more often with colds, and were ill for more than twice as many days.
- In a study at State University of New York in Stony

Brook, 100 healthy adults kept diaries for three months, in which they made notations of all major and minor stresses in their lives, as well as positive events. Each day, they had their saliva studied for secretory IgA. While the positive experiences increased IgA levels for as long as two days, the stressful ones significantly decreased amounts of IgA during the day in which they happened.

· In a study published in 1992 in the journal *Behavioral Medicine,* 17 college students completed a stress questionnaire, and then were infected with a cold virus. Five of the 17 volunteers never developed cold symptoms; these hardy individuals had reported only about one-third as many stressful life events as those who caught colds. The bottom line: Low stress levels seemed to have kept their infection-fighting immune systems strong.

Stress and Your Health

At the University of Washington, Thomas Holmes, M.D., and Richard H. Rahe, M.D., devised a scale of stressful life events that affect health and illness. They ranked these events according to their potential ability to leave an individual susceptible to illnesses, major and minor. Interestingly, while most of the stress-producing circumstances are clearly negative ones (such as death of a close friend or foreclosure on a mortgage), others are usually considered positive (a marriage, Christmas), yet still can be a source of stress.

Here is the life-change scale, with events in descending order of significance in their ability to leave you open to illness:

1. Death of a spouse
2. Divorce
3. Marital separation from mate
4. Detention in jail or other institution
5. Death of a close family member
6. Major personal injury or illness
7. Marriage
8. Being fired at work
9. Marital reconciliation with mate
10. Retirement from work
11. Major change in the health or behavior of a family member
12. Pregnancy
13. Sexual difficulties
14. Gaining a new family member (through birth, adoption, elderly parent moving in, and so on)
15. Major business adjustment (merger, reorganization, bankruptcy, and so on)
16. Major change in financial state (a lot worse off or a lot better off than usual)
17. Death of a close friend
18. Changing to a different line of work
19. Major change in the number of arguments with spouse (either a lot more or a lot less than usual regarding child-rearing, personal habits, and so on)
20. Taking on a mortgage greater than $10,000 (purchasing a house, business, and so on)
21. Foreclosure of a mortgage or loan

22. Major change in responsibilities at work (promotion, demotion, lateral transfer, and so on)
23. Son or daughter leaving home (marriage, attending college, and so on)
24. In-law troubles
25. Outstanding personal achievement
26. Spouse beginning or ceasing work outside the home
27. Beginning or ceasing formal schooling
28. Major change in living conditions (building a new house, remodeling, deterioration of house or neighborhood, and so on)
29. Revision of personal habits (dress, manners, associations, and so on)
30. Troubles with boss
31. Major change in working hours or conditions
32. Change in residence
33. Changing to a new school
34. Major change in usual type and/or amount of recreation
35. Major change in church activities (for example, a lot more or a lot less than usual)
36. Major change in social activities (for example, a lot more or a lot less than usual)
37. Taking on a mortgage or a loan less than $10,000
38. Major change in sleeping habits (a lot more or a lot less sleep, or change in part of day when asleep)
39. Major change in the number of family get-togethers (a lot more or a lot less than usual)
40. Major change in eating habits (a lot more or

a lot less food intake, or very different meal
hours or surroundings)
41. Vacation
42. Christmas
43. Minor violations of the law (traffic tickets, jay-
walking, disturbing the peace, and so on)

COPING WITH STRESS

If you're a "control freak" and climb the walls when
things don't go as you had planned ... or if you have
trouble accepting criticism without fuming inside ... or
if you have difficulty relaxing and enjoying life with
your family and friends—you need to get your stress
levels under control. If you don't, you may be fishing
for handkerchiefs more than most people, while also increasing your vulnerability to even more serious illnesses.

Keep in mind that stressful situations themselves
aren't the real cause for concern; rather, it's the way you
respond to that stress. For some people, being stuck in
traffic isn't a big deal; but others react as though it's the
end of the world. Even if you presently respond to stress
in a frantic, potentially destructive way, however, you
can shift that reaction in a direction that doesn't threaten
your physical well-being.

Part of your own stress-management program might
include improving your communication skills and learning negotiation and assertiveness techniques. You should
also consider learning a relaxation exercise or incorpo-
rating imagery or visualization techniques into your life.

Managing Your Stress More Effectively

Not all stress is easily resolvable. You can't wave a magic wand and put an end to the freeway traffic, for example. If you have a parent who is terminally ill, nothing in your power can change that. But there are ways to cope with any kind of stress more effectively. Here is one approach:

Write down the sources of stress in your life that you *can* change or eliminate from your life. If you're troubled by the "little" things—such as lengthy lines at the bank or unsettling numbers when you step onto the bathroom scale—create a strategy for gaining control of those situations, perhaps by going to the bank during off hours or conscientiously cutting back on the fat in your diet and joining a health club. Write down the changeable sources of stress in your life, and then how you can alleviate them:

1. A source of stress is _____
   _____
   _____

   I can reduce this stress by _____
   _____

2. A source of stress is _____
   _____
   _____

   I can reduce this stress by _____
   _____

3. A source of stress is _____
   _____
   _____

I can reduce this stress by _____
_____

4. A source of stress is _____
_____
_____

I can reduce this stress by _____
_____

Next, write down a list of stresses in your life that you *cannot* change:

1. _____
2. _____
3. _____
4. _____
5. _____

Then decide whether you're willing to accept what isn't changeable, and adopt coping strategies (like the relaxation exercise beginning on the next page) to at least relieve the burden a little and ease the toll it may be taking on your body.

AN ANTIDOTE TO THE FIGHT-OR-FLIGHT RESPONSE

For stress busting, a good place to start is to take a breather—and take it often. Learn a relaxation technique (see the box on page 77), or melt away the anxiety using meditation, imagery, or yoga. Meditation, for example, involves sitting quietly with your eyes closed, and concentrating on a sound, word, or mantra; this process can

relax and calm the body and promote positive physiological changes. When you bring the release of stress
hormones to a screeching halt, your immune function
may improve and muscle tension may subside. "As you
reduce your stress levels, theoretically you should be
able to improve your health," says Barrie Cassilith,
Ph.D., a founding member of the Advisory Council to
the National Institutes of Health's Office of Alternative
Medicine.

Andrew Weil, M.D., the author of *8 Weeks to Optimum Health*, believes that simply connecting with nature
is therapeutic. "Walking or sitting quietly in a natural
setting is a simple form of meditation, an antidote for
being too much in our heads, too focused on thoughts
and emotions," he writes. "If you live in a big city,
seek out a park to visit. You will find the air better there
and the trees comforting. You do not have to do anything in particular, just sit quietly and let the place relax
you."

Recharging with the Relaxation Response

Herbert Benson, M.D., of Harvard Medical School
has estimated that 60 to 90 percent of all visits to the
doctor's office are due to stress-related illnesses. Until he created a technique that he called the Relaxation Response, most Westerners thought that
meditation or relaxation was solely the purview of
yogis or Zen masters.

But then Benson found that the same physiological
benefits could be achieved with a simple exercise.

Here is the technique that Benson devised. Perform it once or twice a day:

1. Sit in a comfortable position in a quiet place.
2. Close your eyes.
3. Relax your muscles.
4. Breathe slowly and naturally. As you do, silently repeat a focus word or a short phrase that you've chosen. It may have a spiritual or religious meaning for you, but it can be any word that you find calming or comforting (for example, it might be *love, peace,* or *om*).
5. Continue to breathe slowly while repeating your word. As you do, maintain a passive attitude. If external thoughts enter your mind (this will inevitably happen), simply say to yourself, "Oh, well," and bring your attention back to your breathing and your focus word.
6. After 10 to 20 minutes, begin to bring the exercise to a close by sitting quietly for another one to two minutes. Next, open your eyes and stay seated for another minute before standing up and going about the rest of your day.

LET YOUR IMAGINATION SOAR

A different relaxation technique involves the use of guided imagery or visualization. This approach, growing in popularity, begins when you enter a state of relaxation; then you call upon your imagination to stimulate the immune system and the healing process.

Perhaps you're familiar with the use of imagery by

cancer patients. Radiation oncologist O. Carl Simonton, M.D., developed an approach in which cancer patients create images of their cancer as broken-up hamburger meat, for example, which is then destroyed by disease-fighting white blood cells in the form of imaginary dogs or white knights on horseback. Or they may form pictures in their mind of a serene setting (perhaps a gorgeous mountain retreat or a beautiful lake), and use this scene to help relax their bodies and soothe their physical pain. Sure, the first time you hear about this kind of imagery, it sounds a little odd, but it is being more widely used as a complement to conventional cancer therapy (for example, chemotherapy or radiation) and other traditional treatments.

Pain specialist David E. Bresler, Ph.D., uses imagery with his patients, often with dramatic results. He relates the story of a woman with chronic and severe facial pain who created a visual image of her mouth "being on fire." With that image in mind, Dr. Bresler suggested that she visualize ways to douse the flames. So the patient pictured the fire being absorbed into cool, floating clouds filled with water. As she practiced this exercise, again and again, the images became stronger, and her pain began to subside.

Martin L. Rossman, M.D., a pioneer in the use of guided imagery to fight disease and the author of *Healing Yourself,* says that you can also use imagery to fight colds and flus. At the end of a relaxation exercise to reduce stress, you can create images of your symptoms, your immune system, and the healing process. According to Dr. Rossman, "If you have trouble creating a personal image, you may want to focus on certain symptoms, such as congestion, and imagine cleansing your

mucous membranes with an antiseptic, decongestant solution. You may also want to imagine your immune cells
as healthy, numerous, active, and effective in eliminating
unwelcome viruses or bacteria from your system.'' He
advises practicing this technique at least twice a day for
15 to 20 minutes each time.

Of 22 studies that have examined whether imagery
can stimulate the immune system, 18 have shown a positive healing connection with diseases ranging from the
common cold to cancer cells. In one widely cited study
at George Washington University and the National Cancer Institute, breast cancer patients practiced imagery,
along with relaxation exercises, for eighteen months;
during that time, their natural killer cell activity increased, as did the responsiveness of their white blood
cells.

Imagery is a powerful means by which the mind can
communicate with the body. By choosing your images
carefully, you may be able to faciliate the healing process. Dr. Bresler says, "If you see yourself as a helpless,
hopeless victim of an illness, your body will probably
respond differently than if you picture yourself as a self-
healing organism.''

STRESS-PROOFING STRATEGIES

No one gets through life without the bangs and bruises
caused by stress. But you can minimize the impact of
that stress—including its ability to weaken your immune
system and leave you vulnerable to colds—with the following techniques:

- *Don't expect perfection,* from either yourself or those around you. If you don't settle for anything less than perfection, you'll never be content; that's because no one ever achieves perfection. Set your goals high, but at attainable levels.
- *Don't overcommit yourself.* Avoid taking on more responsibilities than you can reasonably assume and still keep balance and sanity in your life. If you feel as though you're constantly running in fast-forward, slow down before you burn out. Set priorities. Make some time for play. If you have a job where the stress levels are absolutely impossible and un-changeable, consider finding a new place to work. If you work full-time, and then also have to deal with cooking, cleaning, laundry, bathing the kids, and helping them with homework once you're home—get some help! Sharing the family respon-sibilities or hiring someone to spruce up the house once a week can make all the difference in your world.
- *Express your feelings.* If it's inappropriate to tell off your boss, find another release. Share your feelings with a friend, a family member, or a therapist. Or write them down in a journal. If you keep every-thing inside, your stress levels will soar.
- *Reduce the high-stress components of your life.* If the commute to work is leaving you frazzled, look into car-pooling (it's much more relaxing to read or catch a catnap while someone else is at the wheel dodging the road rage around you).
- *Do something you enjoy each day.* It may simply be spending an hour reading a novel, listening to mu-sic, or getting a massage. It might be going to a

movie, visiting an art museum, or watching a base-
ball game on TV. You need some time just for yourself and your own pleasure.

- *Exercise and eat right.* Regular physical activity can
relieve stress and keep your immune system strong.
A well-balanced diet also can help resist disease.
- *Find the humor in life.* Don't take everything so
seriously. In his book *The Marriage of the Sun and
Moon*, Andrew Weil, M.D., said that he felt tempted
to establish an entire medical-practice system based
on having patients laugh! Some research, in fact,
shows that laughter can strengthen the immune system. But according to Dr. Weil, the average adult
laughs just 17 times a day, compared to 300 times
for the typical 6-year-old.

Here's a sobering study: At Western New England
College in Springfield, Massachusetts, people watched
one of two programs—either an educational video or a
video of a Richard Pryor performance. While the individuals viewing the educational program did not experience any changes in their immune system, as reflected
in measurements of their IgA levels, the group watching Pryor had significant increases in IgA. The bottom
line: At every opportunity, have a good laugh.

- *Get plenty of sleep.* Studies show that just one night
of sleep loss can cause significant declines in natural
killer cells, an important parameter of immune function. If you deprive yourself of sleep, you could be
more susceptible to—and slower to recover from—
colds and flus.
- *Put the stress in your life into perspective.* When

you're anxious over pressures at work, for example, ask yourself, "How important is this going to be in a year (or, for that matter, in a week)?" The circumstances that are driving you crazy today will probably seem insignificant when you look back on them.

KEEPING A STRESS DIARY

You may not even be aware of all the stress in your day-to-day life. Not only is it a good idea to monitor these sources of stress for a while, but also try keeping a record of how you're coping with them. As you become better at managing stress, you'll reduce its impact on your immune system.

For the next two to three weeks, follow these steps:

1. Each night before going to sleep, spend a few minutes reflecting upon your day, and writing down the stress that you encountered.
2. How did you respond to these episodes of stress? Write down how you dealt with them. Did you become angry and upset? Or did you take a deep breath and try to relax?
3. What changes can you make to minimize the recurrence of this stress? Can you respond in a more positive way in the future? Can you eliminate some of the sources of stress? Write down the answers to these questions in each day's diary entries.

AROMATHERAPY: ANOTHER WAY TO RELAX

When you have a cold and your nasal passages are congested, you may feel that your sense of smell has vanished. But believers in aromatherapy say that your olfactory senses are still sharp enough to make you more comfortable and elevate your mood, if not to put a quicker end to the cold itself.

Aromatherapy is extremely popular in Europe and is the most widely used alternative treatment in England. It involves extracting essential oils from the fruit, blossoms, roots, and bark of plants—such as rose, lavender, and chamomile—and dispersing them into the air, putting them in a bath, or rubbing them directly into the skin. Proponents of aromatherapy point out that these oils not only give plants their fragrance, but also have powerful biological properties—so powerful, in fact, that they can change the chemistry within the body and actually influence the disease process. One theory is that these fragrances "turn on" certain receptors in the nasal passages, which in turn transmit information to the limbic region of the brain and influence stress and mood.

Aromatic oils are obtained by heating, steaming, pounding, or soaking the plants in alcohol or hot oil. It takes huge numbers of these plants (dozens and sometimes thousands of pounds of plant material) to produce a single pound of essential oil. But even just a little pleasant fragrance can be used to produce relaxation, ease anxiety, strengthen the immune system, and heal wounds; the claims also extend to halting headaches, easing PMS symptoms, and solving sleep problems.

Of course, we all know that a pleasant odor can have a tranquilizing effect. Smell a rose, and you might quickly forget about everything negative in your life, including the sore throat that has been making you miserable. "When you get a professional massage, there are always some pleasant aromas nearby, which seem to facilitate the relaxation process," says Barrie Cassilith, Ph.D. Researchers working on behalf of shopping-mall and factory owners are investigating which scents—when sent wafting through malls and manufacturing plants—might put consumers in a buying mood and assembly-line workers in a more productive frame of mind!

Where did all of this attachment to aromas get started? Since the Middle Ages, aromatic plants have been used by healers in China, Egypt, and India. But the modern era of "fragrance therapy" dates back to the 1920s in France, where a chemist named René-Maurice Gattefossé was working in the lab of his family's perfume manufacturing company and accidentally burned his hand. Desperately looking for something in which to soak his fiery hand, he submerged it in a vat of pure lavender oil—and became convinced that it had accelerated his healing, and left behind no scar. Gattefossé (and later a group of French physicians) launched a series of studies into the therapeutic properties of aromatic plants; along the way, he created the term *aromatherapy*.

Unfortunately, however, carefully conducted studies into aromatherapy are in short supply. Some research suggests that the scent of lavender accelerates the brain's alpha-wave activity, which appears to be associated with a more relaxed state. Lemon is touted as an immune-system booster, rosemary as an analgesic, and peppermint as a reliever of an upset stomach. Some aromatherapists contend that the best virus-busters and mucus-reducers are geranium, eucalyptus, cinnamon, and sandalwood, while the fastest routes to relaxation use chamomile as well as lavender.

Unlike in Europe, few medical doctors in the United

States are experienced aromatherapists. However, a variety of health-care professionals, including naturopaths (who treat patients without drugs), have begun to incorporate the use of therapeutic fragrances into their practices; health-food stores also sell these essential oils if you want to try a whiff on your own. Put a few drops of oil into a bath, mist it into the air with a diffuser, or place several drops in a bowl of hot water and then inhale the steam to help clear your nasal passages. You can also rub it directly into your skin through massage or via hot or cold compresses. Use small amounts, especially the first time you try a particular oil, if you have a history of allergies. Botanist James Duke, Ph.D., the author of *The Green Pharmacy,* recommends diluting essential oils, perhaps by mixing a few drops with massage lotion or vegetable oil. Most experts advise against ingesting these essential oils by mouth, however, since they could be toxic; according to Dr. Duke, just ½ teaspoon of some formulations can cause death if they're swallowed! If you're pregnant, talk to your obstetrician before trying any of these aromatic oils; some (such as juniper, thyme, and sage) have been associated with causing premature uterine contractions. Read labels of aromatherapy products for storage guidelines. In most cases, they should be kept in a cool location. Some aromatic oils need to be stored in the refrigerator.

Where to Find the Aroma in Aromatherapy

The oils popular in aromatherapy are familiar names and, in many cases, familiar fragrances. The following oils are commonly available in health-food stores:

arnica	jasmine	pine
basil	juniper	rose
bergamot	lavender	rosemary
calamus	lemon	sage
camphor	lily-of-the-valley	sandalwood
chamomile	mandarin	sassafras
cinnamon	marjoram	spearmint
clary sage	melissa	sweet fennel
cloves	myrrh	thyme
cypress	nutmeg	valerian
eucalyptus	orange blossoms	vanilla
everlast	(neroli oil)	vetivert
geranium	palmarosa	wintergreen
grapefruit	peppermint	ylang-ylang

6

A Medley of Complementary Therapies

When a cold or flu epidemic is running rampant through the community, you might be ready to throw in the towel (or at least the Kleenex box) after days of trying to blow away the sniffles. So where do you turn when nothing else seems to work?

In this chapter, we'll review a few complementary (or alternative) therapies worth trying. Your family physician may not be able to tell you much about homeopathy and acupuncture, for example, but the faithful insist that they are the answer for reining in the common cold.

HOMEOPATHY: A LITTLE MEANS A LOT

There's something counterintuitive about homeopathy. After all, for our entire lives we've been told that if one aspirin tablet eases a headache, then two tablets might get rid of it completely. Although one antihypertensive pill a day might not bring your blood pressure down to normal, two pills might.

But according to homeopaths, *less* is better. That's right: extremely small doses of a homeopathic remedy— so small that they can't even be measured!—are exactly what you need to boost your immune system and cure a cold and dozens of other everyday illnesses. The theory is not much different from that of the allergy shots, or immunotherapy, that you might receive from an allergist, in which tiny amounts of an allergy-triggering substance are injected into you, which gradually desensitizes you to that offending material.

Homeopathic potions (available from a practitioner or at a health-food store or pharmacy) are natural substances that are dramatically diluted by mixing them with distilled water and/or alcohol. Most of these healing substances come from plants, minerals, chemicals, and animal products. But the sources of others might make you tremble—for example, some are derived from spiders and bees. Others come from squid ink and poison ivy. The thought of being treated with the remnants of a tarantula might make you content to deal with your cold without any treatment at all. However, what if homeopathy really works?

A Little Background, Please . . .

The George Washington of homeopathy was a medical doctor from Germany named Samuel Hahnemann. He began looking for alternative treatments in an era when physicians had evaluated therapies such as bloodletting and purging on the front lines of healing.

Hahnemann developed a theory that, to most mainstream doctors, still seems on the fringe. It proclaimed that the best way to treat a disease is to give very small doses of the precise substance that caused it in the first place; in other words, the best remedy for any ailment is tiny amounts of what produces the same symptoms that you're trying to relieve. When taken in infinitesimal doses, they can stimulate the immune system, according to Hahnemann, whether the problem is a sore throat or something more serious. Hahnemann labeled this philosophy of medicine "like cures like," or the "law of similars." The word *homeopathy* was drawn from the Greek words *homoios*, meaning "like," and *pathos*, meaning "suffering". The underlying concept may not have been new at all; in 400 B.C., Hippocrates wrote that illness is cured through "application of the like."

The Art of Dilution

When you think about dilution, you might imagine a ratio of ten to one, or even a hundred to one—but not when you're talking about homeopathy. In homeopathic medicines, the ratio is absolutely mind-boggling: one drop of the active substance, mixed with a hundred thousand—or even a million—drops of water! Companies that produce these products perform dilutions in a serial manner—that is, they dilute a solution ten times, then take a portion of that dilution, and dilute it ten more times, and then repeat the process again and again. Hahnemann called this phenomenon the "law of infinitesimals," proclaiming that the greater the dilution, the more powerful the potion. It has become the foundation on which homeopathy is based.

No wonder skeptics of homeopathy abound. After all,

because of the extreme dilutions, some remedies do not contain *any* molecules of the initial substance! That's right, none. Barrie Cassilith, Ph.D., the author of *The Alternative Medicine Handbook,* points out, "The doses are not minute! They're non-existent! When there's less than a molecule, there's nothing there!" Homeopathic claims, say critics, run counter to simple laws of chemistry and pharmacology. But don't tell that to the homeopaths. They insist that rhythmic shaking of the potion reinvigorates or "potentizes" the mixture with its own "vital force," and reactivates a "trace memory," an "imprint" or a "pattern" of the active ingredient in the liquid, which resonates and produces therapeutic effects. Some homeopaths believe that an electromagnetic energy is associated with the remedy's active ingredient, and even when this ingredient can no longer be detected and measured, the energy is still at work, however subtly.

Sound far-fetched? Can liquids have memories? Well, many modern French physicians—about one-third of them, in fact—have incorporated homeopathy into their practices, and obviously find value in it, although the reasons for its efficacy remain something of a mystery to most scientists. In the United Kingdom, the national health-insurance plan covers homeopathic treatments. In the United States, homeopathy is practiced by some medical doctors, as well as by chiropractors, homeopaths, osteopaths, dentists, and other health-care professionals. "Homeopathic doctors say that traditional physicians use powerful medications to suppress diseases, and thus interfere with the body's own natural healing abilities," says George A. Ulett, M.D., Ph.D., the author of *Alternative Medicine or Magical Healing.*

Although a number of studies have examined the efficacy of homeopathy, few have looked specifically at the common cold and influenza. Nevertheless, the overall value of homeopathy has been supported by research published in prestigious medical journals such as *The Lancet*. Wayne Jonas, M.D., director of the National Institutes of Health's Office of Alternative Medicine, took up the challenge of determining whether there really was something to this therapy that features "nothing." He and his colleagues evaluated 89 existing placebo-controlled studies of homeopathy, conducted between 1943 and 1995, and collectively evaluated them in a so-called meta-analysis; in essence, they created one huge study using all of the data from these many studies. Their conclusion: There's more to homeopathy than something imaginary. In their research, homeopathic remedies were about two-and-a-half times more likely to have a positive effect on illness than a placebo. When Dr. Jonas and his co-investigators limited their analysis to the 26 best-designed studies, homeopathy still showed statistically significant benefits (although to a lesser degree). They wrote, "The results of our meta-analysis are not compatible with the hypothesis that the clinical effects of homeopathy are completely due to a placebo." They urged more research into homeopathy, despite what they deemed "its implausibility."

There is other good news in all of this: Because homeopathic portions are so diluted, they are virtually risk-free. Consuming a homeopathic remedy is like drinking a glass of water. At best, it will bring a quicker end to your cold or flu; at worst, it will supply some of the fluids you should be consuming anyway when you're ill.

Calming a Cold

David E. Bresler, Ph.D., of the UCLA School of Medicine, says that a full-out assault on a cold could include homeopathic treatments—and more. For example, he might try a homeopathic remedy called *Natrum mur*, which is designed to relieve coughing and sneezing; he'll back it up with plenty of fluids, lots of vitamins and minerals, and acupuncture treatments.

There are literally thousands of homeopathic remedies available, for virtually everything that ails you. Most of them have names that sound like they're out of a foreign-language dictionary. For the common cold, practitioners might recommend remedies such as *Nux vomica, Bryonia alba, Ferrum phoshoricum, Allium cepa,* and *Euphrasia*. Others might choose *Belladonna,* obtained from a flowering but poisonous plant called nightshade; at full strength, the plant can cause flu-like symptoms such as a fever, but at infinitesimal homeopathic doses, the hope is that it can cure the flu.

In Dr. Jonas's book *Healing with Homeopathy,* he lists several homeopathic medicines that are most useful for the common cold, and he advises taking the remedy you choose two to four times a day (depending on the potency) for two to three days. *Ferrum phosphoricum,* he says, is most useful in the early stages of the common cold, when symptoms include a slight fever and a feeling of lethargy. *Kali iodatum* is particularly useful when your nose is running like a faucet and you have a headache between the eyes. Other homeopathic remedies he recommends include *Aconitum napellus, Pulsatilla, Allium cepa, Arsenicum album, Euphrasia, Mercurius vivus,* and *Nux vomica*.

The most popular remedy for influenza has an absolutely impossible-to-remember name—*Oscillococcinum* (try saying it three times fast—or even once!). But after you read about its origin, you might instinctively feel that it's not for you. *Oscillococcinum* comes from duck hearts and livers, which, according to homeopathic practitioners, contain infinitesimal amounts of flu virus antibodies, and thus can combat the flu in humans. According to Dr. Jonas, it has been ''scientifically shown to hasten recovery in patients with influenza when compared to placebo.'' It's probably worth trying, and certainly safe, and should be taken when the first symptoms of colds, flus, or sore throats appear. Some practitioners recommend a dose of *Oscillococcinum* once a week throughout cold and flu season to keep the bugs at bay. But the dilutions of *Oscillococcinum* are absolutely mind-boggling. In fact, a University of Maryland physicist put his computer to work and calculated that the odds of consuming even one molecule of duck liver or heart in a potion of *Oscillococcinum* are less than those of being struck by an asteroid!

As for other flu remedies, Dr. Jonas recommends *Gelsemium* (when you feel dull and listless, and your face is flushed), *Bryonia alba* (when you have the chills and are extremely thirsty), and *Eupatorium perfoliatum* (for aching muscles and bones).

What Do All Those Names Mean?

The names of most homeopathic remedies are enough to drive you a little crazy. But if you can get beyond them, these treatments don't seem all that mysterious after all. Here are the Latin names of some of the more common potions you're likely to encounter, and their English translations or equivalent:

Aconitum napellus	monkshood
Allium cepa	red onion
Amica	mountain daisy
Apis mellifica	crushed bee
Argentum metallicum	silver
Arsenicum album	trioxide of arsenic
Arum tryphyllum	Indian turnip
Baptisa tinctoria	wild indigo
Belladonna	deadly nightshade
Bryonia alba	wild hops
Calcarea carbonica	oyster shell
Calendula	marigold
Cantharis	Spanish fly
Capsicum	chili pepper
Chamomilla	German chamomile

Coffea cruda	unroasted coffee bean
Colocynthis	bitter cucumber
Conium maculatum	hemlock
Cuprum metallicum	copper
Dioscorea villosa	wild yam
Eupatorium perfoliatum	thoroughwort
Euphrasia	eyebright
Ferrum phosphoricum	phosphate of iron
Gelsemium sempervirens	yellow jasmine
Hamamelis	witchhazel
Iodum	iodine
Kali iodatum	iodide of potassium
Lachesis	venom of bushmaster snake
Ledum palustre	labrador tea
Mercurius vivus	quicksilver
Mezereum	spurge olive
Natrum mur	salt
Nux vomica	poison nut
Oscillococcinum	duck heart, liver
Pulsatilla	windflower

Ranunculus bulbosus	bulbous butter-cup
Rhus toxicodendron	poison ivy
Sepia	cuttlefish
Spongia tosta	roasted sea sponge

Homeopathic remedies are available as liquid drops and capsules. Although you can self-prescribe those that are sold at health-food stores, a homeopathic physician can personalize the treatment for you. Most homeopathic practitioners (there are about 3,000 in the United States, trained through the National Center for Homeopathy) might spend an hour or more with you during your first visit, finding out as much as possible about the whole person they're treating so they can customize the therapy; a practitioner may tell you, "I'm not treating the flu; I'm treating an individual who has the flu."

For more information about homeopathic remedies, contact the National Center for Homeopathy (801 N. Fairfax St., Suite 306, Alexandria, VA 22314).

ACUPUNCTURE: GETTING TO THE POINT—OR PURE BUNK?

If you still have chilling flashbacks about the vaccinations you got as a child to protect you from pediatric diseases, your last choice for stopping the flow of the common cold or the flu might be to volunteer to be jabbed and stabbed with needles—with the hope of making you feel better! It's an understandable reaction. But many people believe that acupuncture can make a difference.

In the early 1970s, most Americans had never heard of acupuncture. But after Richard Nixon's trip to China, it gradually built up a following in the United States. Thousands of acupuncturists now have been trained and practice here, and this ancient health-care modality has gained respectability throughout America. Although it is used primarily to treat pain (including headaches and back pain)—with studies showing that it can relieve pain in 55 to 85 percent of patients—it has also helped people with a wide range of health problems ranging from insomnia to asthma. And by keeping the body in balance, it may be able to prevent or quickly resolve the common cold.

During a typical acupuncture treatment, a series of very thin, metallic needles (typically, up to ten or twelve of them) are inserted into specific acupuncture points, after a little rubbing alcohol is applied to each site. You might feel a mild pinch, stinging, or tingling when each needle is inserted; some patients have compared it to the sensation of a mosquito bite. Once these needles are gently tapped into place (typically to a depth of as much as 1 inch), they may be turned, twirled, or in some cases stimulated with electrical currents. An average treatment lasts for 15 to 30 minutes, occasionally longer.

Sometimes, to strengthen the effects of acupuncture, practitioners may add a procedure called *moxabustion* to the acupuncture mix. ''They burn a substance called wormwood, either right on the needle itself, or on some ginger root that is placed on the skin,'' says George A. Ulett, M.D., Ph.D., a pioneering acupuncture researcher. Some practitioners also intensify the benefits with the use of sound waves.

No one knows for sure how acupuncture works for the common cold or for anything else (see the adjoining box). But that hasn't kept Americans from getting the point that, in some cases, acupuncture can improve their health. No wonder the FDA estimates that up to twelve million acupuncture treatments are performed in the United States each year. The World Health Organization's list of about 40 ailments treatable with acupuncture include the common cold and sinusitis.

How Does Acupuncture Work?

There's nothing new about acupuncture. Its history dates back at least 2,500 years. But investigators trying to describe how this fine art of needling works often become stuck for an explanation.

Ask the Chinese how acupuncture works, and they'll probably describe the opposing forces (*yin* and *yang*) that flow through the body, moving along a road map of fourteen pathways called *meridians*. If these forces are out of balance, and one of these meridians becomes blocked, you're no longer going with the flow (so to speak), and you may become ill.

But acupuncture can come to the rescue. All of the 362 traditional acupuncture points lie along the meridians, and by inserting needles at several of these sites, the energy flow of the body can be brought into balance by altering the vital life force called *qi* (pronounced "chee").

This concept runs so counter to Western thinking that scientists in the United States and elsewhere have sought some alternate explanation for the efficacy of acupuncture. One hypothesis is that meridians coincide with neural pathways, but this theory hasn't panned out.

"The hypothesis that is most understandable to the Western mind is that acupuncture stimulates the body's natural morphinelike substances, called endorphins, which may help explain acupuncture's painkilling properties," says Victor Sierpina, M.D., assistant professor of family medicine at the University of Texas Medical Branch in Galveston. Other theories suggest that the needles stimulate the release of various hormones and neurotransmitters.

In 1997, an expert panel convened by the National Institutes of Health concluded that there was "clear evidence" of acupuncture's efficacy in several areas, including reducing postoperative dental pain and minimizing nausea associated with surgery, chemotherapy, and pregnancy. The credibility of that report could free up more research funds to investigate other areas for which acupuncture is commonly used.

If you're treated by a trained practitioner, acupuncture is safe and effective. On rare occasions, a needle may break, an organ (for example, a lung or the bladder) might be punctured, and the patient may experience bleeding. But these problems are much more the exception than the rule, and are very uncommon in trained hands. Because needles should be sterilized and discarded after a single use, infections are rare.

If you decide to try acupuncture, here are some tips to keep in mind:

- There are about 7,000 health-care professionals in the United States who are also licensed acupuncturists; however, not every state requires licensing of acupuncturists. Look for a practitioner certified by the National Commission for the Certification of Acupuncturists (your own family physician may be able to provide you with a referral). Degrees or titles such as C.A. (Certified Acupuncturist) or L.Ac. (Licensed Acupuncturist) are granted by state licensing boards.
- A single acupuncture treatment may be helpful if you suffer from a cold or the flu. But for a more chronic condition, you will probably need a series of ten or more treatments.
- For the names of acupuncturists in your community, contact the American Association of Oriental Medicine (433 Front St., Catasauqua, PA 18032; phone: 610-433-2448).

Acupuncture: Good for What Ails You?

The common cold and the flu are only two illnesses that can be treated with acupuncture. Here are some other ailments that acupuncturists frequently treat with this ancient modality:

allergies	depression	menopausal
anxiety	diarrhea	symptoms
arthritis	drug addiction	neck pain
asthma	fibromyalgia	premenstrual
back pain	(general	syndrome (PMS)
bronchitis	muscular	sciatica
bursitis	pain)	shoulder pain
carpal	headaches	sinusitis
tunnel	hypertension	stress
syndrome	(high blood	stroke
chronic	pressure)	rehabilitation
fatigue	impotence	tendinitis
constipation	insomnia	vertigo
cough	knee pain	(dizziness)

JUICING AND FASTING: LIVING THE LIQUID LIFE

The world of complementary and alternative medicine is replete with all kinds of therapies, each with its own following. Juicing is one of the more popular. You've probably seen the infomercials on late-night television proclaiming that drinking the juices of every conceivable type of fresh fruit and vegetable can keep you disease-free. Buy and use one of their juicers, they proclaim, and good health is all but guaranteed.

Of course, the vitamins, minerals, and other nutrients in juices can help boost the immune system, and some of them (most notably vitamin C) have been associated with cold busting. Through juicing, you're getting these nutrients in a raw, concentrated form that can pack a real health-promoting wallop. So the more of these juices you drink before or while you're ill, the better. But juice consumption is often undertaken in conjunction with liquid fasts, and fasting may not be the best option when you're fighting an infection like a cold or the flu.

If you decide to try fasting and relying on juice (or tea) as your sole source of nourishment, do so only under a physician's guidance. Proponents of fasting insist that once you free the body from the task of breaking down food for digestion, it will be able to direct more of its energies toward recovering from illness. True, short fasts (one to two days) are probably not going to do any harm, but if you go beyond that, you could be asking for trouble, particularly if your immune system is already working overtime to battle the flu or another illness.

"The research shows that fasting not only doesn't boost the immune system, but it actually interferes with immune function," insists Barrie Cassilith, Ph.D. While some people report feeling spiritual benefits from fasting, you might be advised to reserve fasting for times when you're not fighting a short-term infection (although proponents insist that food avoidance promotes a detoxification and cleansing process).

What Nutrients Can Juices Provide?

No doubt about it: Fresh fruits and vegetables are excellent sources of vitamins and minerals. Here is where to find some of the most important vitamins and minerals that play a role in strengthening the immune system and, in turn, fighting off viruses:

Beta-carotene/vitamin A	Apricots, asparagus, broccoli, cantaloupe, carrots, celery, guavas, kale, mangoes, nectarines, peaches, spinach, sweet potatoes, tangerines, tomatoes
Folic acid	Asparagus, bananas, broccoli, butternut squash, cauliflower, grapefruit juice, green beans, lima beans, oranges, potatoes, spinach, squash,

	sweet potatoes, tomatoes
Selenium	Apricots, carrots, celery, grape-fruit, mush-rooms, onions, oranges, turnips
Vitamin B_6	Bananas, carrots, figs, kidney beans, lima beans, pineapple, potatoes, spin-ach, sweet pota-toes, tomatoes, turnip greens
Vitamin C	Acorn squash, broccoli, brus-sels sprouts, cab-bage, cantaloupe, cauliflower, grapefruit, green peas, guavas, honeydew melon, kale, lemons, man-goes, oranges, papayas, pep-pers, pineapple, potatoes, straw-berries, sweet potatoes

Vitamin E	Apricots, asparagus, blueberries, kale, green peas, lima beans, mangoes, olives, peaches, soybeans, sweet potatoes
Zinc	Black-eyed peas, carrots, lima beans, pinto beans

7

A Cold-Free Lifestyle

So how do you chase away a cold? Bernard Macfadden, an eccentric fitness fanatic in the 1920s, was convinced that he had the solution. His plan was spelled out in a book, *Colds, Coughs and Catarrh,* and was founded on his belief that poisons in the body are responsible for colds. His therapeutic regimen included meals that consisted solely of oranges and water, regular naked outdoor "air baths," and a daily enema. He also advised wrapping cold, wet sheets around the head and throat, insisting that this approach was a "powerful eliminator." Colds could be avoided, he insisted, by not gossiping and by going to bargain-basement sales (no explanation as to why was ever offered).

Fortunately, Macfadden didn't have the last word on preventing and caring for colds. Perhaps he had the right idea, though, in paying attention to lifestyle (although he did appear to lose his direction a bit). In your own efforts to evade colds, there are ways to keep your defenses strong—without having to resort to air baths or enemas. In this chapter, let's discuss some simple, sensible lifestyle changes you can make.

KEEP YOUR HANDS CLEAN

In the Academy Award–winning movie *As Good As It Gets,* Jack Nicholson's character, Melvin, was so afraid of germs that his medicine cabinet was crammed with Neutrogena soap. Each time he washed his hands, he would open a new bar, lather up, rinse, and then throw it away after a single use. There were dozens more awaiting his next trip to the sink.

Sure, Melvin was a cleanliness freak. But at the other extreme, most Americans don't wash their hands as often as they should. If they were a little more conscientious about keeping their hands clean, they would probably need the Kleenex box less often.

A 1997 study at Purdue University evaluated the hand-cleansing habits of children and the number of days they missed school because of illness. Those youngsters who washed their hands four or more times a day had 24 percent fewer absences due to colds and flu, and 50 percent fewer days lost because of intestinal illnesses, than children who washed less frequently.

The key times to head for the sink and the soap are before preparing meals or eating, after using the toilet, after sneezing or coughing, and before you touch your eyes, nose, or mouth. And when you do wash your hands, no quick rinses, please! Spend a minute or two doing a thorough job, including lathering up the front *and* back of your hands and washing between your fingers and under your nails. Viruses are hardy critters, and if you rush through the process, you may be doing little more than moving the viruses from one part of your hands to another. Make sure you use soap and hot water, and get a little friction going as you rub your hands together and then use a clean towel.

GET MOVING!

"No pain, no gain!" Well, not exactly. You don't have to exercise to the point of pain and exhaustion. But regular, vigorous exercise can awaken your immune system and keep your body as free of colds as possible.

Humorist Robert Benchley had another vision, however. In writing about ways to avoid the common cold, he advised *eliminating* exercise from your life. "Exercise just stirs up the poisons in your system and makes you a hot-bed of disease," he said. "Sit, or lie, as still as possible and smoke constantly."

Interesting advice. If only Benchley had known that when you take a brisk walk or swim a few laps, you almost immediately increase your arsenal of infection-fighting white blood cells—the Green Berets of your immune system. A study at Appalachian State University in Boone, North Carolina, found that when women in their thirties took brisk walks for 45 minutes five days a week, they had colds for only five days during the fifteen-week study, compared to ten days of colds in a group that never exercised. A separate study by the same researchers reached similar conclusions for women in their sixties, seventies, and eighties; those women who walked an average of 37 minutes a day, five days a week, had less than half as many colds as a sedentary group.

So if the only exercise you're getting these days is punching the buttons on your TV's remote control device, add a little more activity to your life. A brisk walk for 30 minutes, three to four times a week, can put your immune system into overdrive. There's no need to go to extremes; in fact, if you work out at an intense level for over an hour, the positive benefits of exercise start to be overtaken by the negative effects of the fatigue factor. Your immune system will actually start to implode when you overdo it.

Walking may be the ideal exercise. You can do it just about anywhere, its only cost is the price of a good pair of walking shoes, and it's virtually risk-free in terms of injuries. Walking not only helps fight off infections, but it's also good for your heart, lowering your blood pressure and cholesterol level. It also can ease depression, preserve bone strength, and perhaps even fight off some forms of cancer.

Should you forget about exercise when you're under the weather? You may have heard that you can "sweat out" or "run off" a cold by exercising through the sniffles, but that's only a myth. A little exercise-driven perspiration isn't going to make you recover more quickly— nor is it going to slow down your recovery. A study at Ball State University in Muncie, Indiana, found that students with colds had similar illness durations, and the severity of their colds was identical, whether they exercised or rested while sick.

If you don't have a fever, and if your cold is confined to your nose and throat (and hasn't found a home in your chest), there's no reason to become a couch potato until your symptoms disappear. However, if you feel absolutely lousy—your muscles ache and you feel run-down and on fire—give yourself a break for a few days. Let your fever subside (exercise will only send it higher) before lacing up your walking shoes again.

CRUSH OUT YOUR CIGARETTES

When you hear the slogan, "Cigarette smoking may be hazardous to your health," a lot of diseases—most notably cancer and heart disease—probably come to mind before the common cold. But, in fact, if you need yet another reason to give up cigarettes, the link between smoking and colds may be the proverbial straw that breaks the camel's back. If you are a smoker, you will probably get more colds—and colds that are more severe—than a nonsmoker.

"Smoking paralyzes the cilia, the tiny hairs that line the respiratory tract that help clear away viruses and other organisms," says infectious-diseases specialist Steven Mostow, M.D. If these protective cilia aren't doing their job, sweeping away germs that are sneaking around the breathing passages, colds are much more likely to develop. One report concluded that a single cigarette can disable the cilia for up to 30 to 40 minutes. Smoking may also hobble the immune system and increase the inflammatory response—still more good reasons to say good-bye to cigarettes.

In 1993, researchers at Carnegie Mellon University in Pittsburgh joined with investigators at the Common Cold Unit in Salisbury, England, to investigate the possible link between cigarette smoking and colds. In their study, 417 healthy men and women (ages 18 to 54) underwent medical exams and lab tests and answered questionnaires about their smoking and other lifestyle habits. Then they were deliberately exposed to either a cold virus or a saline solution, both via nasal drops; the volunteers remained in a quarantine setting for seven days. In the group of volunteers receiving the actual virus, the nonsmokers were more resistant to catching colds; the smokers were twice as likely to develop a cold as the nonsmokers.

One other finding from the study was particularly surprising: The nonsmokers who were also drinkers of alcohol were even more likely to remain cold-free—and the more they drank (up to three or four drinks a day), the stronger the knockout blow against the cold virus. For example, the nonsmokers who consumed one to two drinks a day had about a 65 percent lower risk of catching a cold than abstainers; the risk was about 85 percent lower in those having two to three drinks a day. This apparent protective effect of alcohol occurred only in the nonsmokers, however.

Just how might alcohol fight off the cold virus? Read on . . .

THE BENEFITS OF DRINKING

Sir William Osler, one of the great teachers and innovators in U.S. and Canadian medical history, once offered the following advice about how to deal with a cold: "Go to bed. Put a hat on the bedpost. Drink whiskey until you see two hats."

Researchers have traditionally felt that alcohol impairs the human immune system; however, most studies pointing in that direction have been conducted with heavy drinkers. If you're consuming more moderate amounts, alcohol could become an ally in keeping you healthy.

How do a couple of drinks bolster your resistance to the common cold, as in the Carnegie Mellon study? Some investigators believe that modest amounts of alcohol interfere with the cold virus's ability to replicate by strengthening the immune response. Others hypothesize that alcohol has an anti-inflammatory effect on the mucous membranes in the nasal passages, and thus minimizes cold symptoms. While alcohol abuse can impair the immune system, a moderate intake may be just what the doctor ordered.

Of course, no one is recommending that people take up drinking as a way to stay cold-free. This may be an intoxicating concept, but there are better strategies than this one. Also, keep in mind that while moderate drinking seems to support heart hardiness (by boosting the "good" HDL cholesterol and interfering with blood clots), recent research shows that even modest amounts of alcohol appear to raise the risk of breast cancer in women (and perhaps cancers of the lung, esophagus, and pancreas). Once you add the greater chance of liver damage and the increased likelihood of automobile accidents associated with alcohol intake, drinking may be too much of a risk in your efforts to keep colds at a distance.

Nevertheless, if you enjoy having an occasional glass or two of wine with dinner, go ahead. Your heart may thank you, and perhaps you'll drive away the cold bugs in the process.

Alcohol: It's Not for Everyone

Although moderate alcohol consumption has several clear benefits, some people should *never* drink. If you answer yes to any of the following questions, stay away from alcohol altogether (or talk to your physician before you take a drink):

- Are you pregnant or trying to become pregnant?
- Are you breast-feeding?
- Do you have high blood pressure that is uncontrolled?
- Do you experience arrhythmias (irregular heart rhythms)?
- Do you have liver disease?
- Do you have peptic ulcers?
- Do you take medications that can interact with alcohol? These drugs include amphetamines, tricyclic antidepressants, meperidine (Demerol), methotrexate, MAO inhibitors, and sleep-inducing drugs, among others; discuss the medications you're taking with your physician for possible alcohol interactions. **Never mix alcohol with cold medications you might be taking, since they can create a severe depressive state**.
- Are you an alcoholic, or have you been treated for alcohol abuse?

YOU GOTTA HAVE FRIENDS

Since you can catch the common cold from the people around you, common sense suggests that the less human contact you have, the better. And while that certainly makes sense when your friends or co-workers are coughing up a storm, nurturing friends and family members can generally provide a cold-proofing shield of armor.

That was the conclusion of a study in 1997 by cold researchers at Carnegie Mellon University. They evaluated 276 people (ages 18 to 55), and examined the scope and variety of their social circles (spouse, children, other relatives, friends, co-workers, neighbors, contacts in social and religious organizations). In their analysis, the investigators controlled for other factors that might contribute to an individual's susceptibility to catching colds, such as stress, low vitamin C consumption, cigarette smoking, and sleep loss.

Then the volunteers were deliberately exposed to rhinoviruses (given through nose drops) and were monitored over a five-day period for signs of a cold. Those people who tended to be the most socially isolated (three or fewer types of social relationships) had four times the risk of catching colds of those with plenty of social ties (six or more types of relationships). Even when the social butterflies did get colds, their symptoms tended to be milder.

Why are colds less common among the gregarious than the reclusive? Carnegie Mellon psychologist Sheldon Cohen, Ph.D., believes that friendly folks with plenty of social support tend to have less anxiety, depression, and other psychological distress. They are more likely to weather the storm of day-to-day stress when they feel the comfort of caring people in their lives. As a result, their immune systems tend to remain stronger and less vulnerable to a sneak attack by cold germs. These neighborly people also are often happier with their lives, and their higher self-worth translates into taking better care of themselves in many different ways: they may be less likely to smoke, for example, or they may get plenty of sleep.

This study supports a substantial and growing body of research showing that companionship is good for your health. Perhaps the most classic of these studies was conducted by Lisa Berkman and Leonard Syme at the University of California, Berkeley, who evaluated residents of Alameda County, California, over a nine-year period to determine whether a relationship exists between social connectedness and life expectancy. Berkman and Syme concluded that people with the fewest social ties had twice the risk of dying as those with the most social connections. In some categories, the risks were even more startling; for example, for every socially active woman beween ages 30 and 49 who died, 4.6 socially inactive women died.

A separate study at the University of California involved cancer patients and looked at the number of social contacts they had on a typical day. Women with the lowest number of social contacts had more than twice the risk of dying of their cancer over a seventeen-year period, compared to women with the greatest number of contacts.

The bottom line: Take time to nurture your family relationships and friendships. One of the payoffs may be a stronger immune system and a greater ability to vanquish cold viruses. As Dr. Cohen said, "Telling people to reduce stress and enjoy the support of their friends, family, and their peers is never a bad thing."

A GOLD MINE OF COLD-COMBAT TIPS

There are other ways to reduce your cold risks—or to blast your way through a viral attack if a cold does strike. Here are some tips on how to arm yourself for battle:

Sleep, Glorious Sleep

Robert Benchley had it right when he advised his readers to make sure they were well rested when combating colds. He wrote, "Get plenty of sleep. If you feel drowsy at your work, just put your head over on your desk and take a little nap. Your boss will understand if you put a little sign up by your elbow reading: 'Man asleep here. Cold prevention.' "

If you're one of those people who also put their heads on their pillows at night and don't budge for eight hours, you could be cutting down your risk of catching a cold even further. Benchley was right; the immune system needs some R & R to recuperate for the next day's battles, and by getting seven to eight hours of sleep a night, you'll be equipped to wage war with cold viruses and other microbial stealth bombers.

If you happen to catch a cold, getting adequate rest is equally important. But that doesn't necessarily mean crawling into bed for days until your symptoms subside. Bed rest isn't going to cure a cold. Getting on with your normal, daily activities is fine, as long as you feel up to it, you don't have a fever, your muscles don't ache, and you don't feel weak and worn to a frazzle. At the same time, listen to your body and don't push yourself; just give in if your body is telling you to slow down for a

day or two. Do whatever you need to heal and regain
strength.

By the way, as a people, Americans are notoriously
sleep deprived. While the average adult needs seven to
eight hours a night, many get only five or six, and drag
themselves through the next day. As their sleep debt
accumulates, night after night, their immune systems become a little weaker in fighting the bugs that cause colds
and more serious illnesses.

Good Hydration

You've heard it for years: When you're sick, drink fluids—and then drink more of them. You can start with
chicken soup (see page 27), but it shouldn't end there.
For many people, a cold-fighting day wouldn't be complete without hot water with lemon and/or honey; for
others, it might be several cups of herbal tea, vegetable
or fruit juice, club soda, or mineral water. Just about any
kind of fluid can ease congestion by moistening and
thinning your nasal secretions (a few fluids should be
avoided; see the adjoining box). Liquids can also loosen
the phlegm in your breathing passages and make coughs
more productive. They can prevent dehydration, too.
And when you're not downing another glass of liquid,
keep your throat moist by sucking on hard candy or
throat lozenges.

By the way, some doctors recommend perching a
glass of water by your bedside. A few sips if you awaken
during the night will help relieve congestion and make
sleeping easier.

And what about prevention? When you're cold-free
and want to stay that way, eight glasses of fluids a day
may be part of the answer. They help keep the mucous

membranes lining the respiratory tract strong, lubricated, and ready to capture surreptitious viruses trying to gain a foothold for their cloak-and-dagger work.

Fluids: Are Some Taboo?

As important as fluids are to your comfort and recovery from colds and flus, there are some you should avoid. Stay away from caffeinated beverages, for example, as well as sugar-laden drinks, when you're battling a cold. And while alcohol may have some benefits in keeping colds at bay, there are some more solidly proven choices when the germs have already taken hold.

Nevertheless, some over-the-counter cold and flu medications actually contain alcohol. That's the case with products such as Vicks NyQuil Liquid, Comtrex Maximum Strength Liquid, and Vicks 44M Cough, Cold & Flu Relief. Many physicians advise caution when using medications that contain alcohol.

Keep It Humid

To give your respiratory tract an extra burst of moisture when you're under the weather, run a cool-mist humidifier in your home. It will keep your mucous membranes from being hung out to dry, and can make you more comfortable. The high humidity will loosen phlegm while soothing a gravelly throat.

Use a humidity gauge to help you keep track of the water content of the air. A portable humidifier should maintain humidity levels at 30 to 50 percent. Also, set the thermostat of your home's heating system low, particularly at night, since heated air will tend to lower the indoor humidity.

Be sure to clean your humidifier daily (follow manufacturer's instructions, which may include using diluted bleach, and then rinsing thoroughly); bacteria and mold can take up residence in a dirty humidifier. Bacteria spewed into the air could cause other infectious diseases, and mold may trigger an allergy-driven runny nose and sneezing to compete with your existing cold symptoms.

In recent years, some doctors have theorized that inhaling hot steam can be a definitive treatment for the common cold. They have theorized that steam can not only ease symptoms, but also increase the temperature in the nasal passages to a level that blocks replication of the cold virus. Initial studies in the 1980s proved promising; an Israeli study found milder cold symptoms in volunteers who inhaled hot steam, compared to those breathing moist air at room temperature. In light of research like this, one medical journal article carried the headline "Hot News on the Common Cold." However, more recent studies haven't found the same positive effects. In one of them, in which patients with colds received 30-minute intranasal treatments of humidified air, the steam had no effect on the replication of rhinoviruses; others have found no improvement of symptoms. A 1994 editorial in the *Journal of the American Medical Association* concluded, "We now bring another rhinovirus saga, which started so positively, to a close and must throw cold water on previous hot news."

Nevertheless, many cold sufferers find that spending a few extra minutes in a hot shower or bath keeps their nasal passages moist and makes them feel better. If that happens with you, turn on the hot water and enjoy!

Back to School: When Is It OK?

Colds are contagious in the 24 hours immediately preceding the onset of symptoms, and then during the first day or two when symptoms are present. That means that your child does not have to remain home from school during the entire seven-to-ten-day course of his cold, but only during the period when he might infect others, or when he simply isn't feeling well. After the period of contagion has passed, he can return to school even with a runny or stuffy nose or with a minor headache.

According to the American Academy of Pediatrics, you can send your child to school unless she meets any of the following criteria. She should remain home when:

- she is running a fever;
- she does not feel well enough to concentrate and participate in class; or
- you think she might be contagious to her classmates.

If you have a baby or a toddler in day care, and you're unable to stay home with him when he has a cold, make sure the staff members know of his illness so they can keep him away from other youngsters as much as possible during the time when he may still be contagious.

By the way, middle-ear infections are *not* contagious. Thus, if your youngster has an ear infection but her fever and pain have subsided, she can go back to school.

The Fine Art of Gargling

When a scratchy throat is making you miserable, soothe it by gargling with warm salt water. Sure, you can splurge on a commercial gargle, but most doctors concede that it carries no advantage over the home remedy.

Preparing a potion for gargling is quick and simple: Stir ¼ to ½ teaspoon of salt into 8 ounces of warm water. A sugar-water gargle is another option: Mix 1 tablespoon of Karo syrup with 8 ounces of water, and use it as you would any other gargle.

Nice and Easy Does It

What could be simpler than blowing your nose? All of us have been doing it since childhood, yet there are plenty of myths surrounding it. Some people believe that you can actually burst an eardrum if you honk your horn too hard. Not true. Yes, you may feel some vibrations and other sensations in your ears as you're blowing, but those are caused by pressure changes that can't rupture the eardrum. However, when you blow very hard, it's possible to strain and break a blood vessel or two in your already tender and fragile nose, but this bleeding should not last for more than a minute or two. Another risk is blowing your nose so hard that the pressure sends infected mucus from the nose into the ear, where it can contribute to the development of a middle-ear infection.

What's the best way to blow your nose? Exhale gently through both nostrils at the same time. Some people press on their nose so that both nostrils are almost closed while they blow; but they won't clear their nose this way, and it's more likely to propel mucus into the ears. No matter what technique you use, avoid high-pressure blowing, please.

Children in particular tend to sniff runny secretions back up into their nose as they try to make it easier to breathe. Once this behavior becomes a habit, however, it can last a lifetime. Teach your child the proper way to blow his or her nose with a tissue (a sleeve is a poor second choice!).

Give Your Toothbrush the Brush-Off

After you've gotten over a cold or the flu, toss out your toothbrush and replace it with a new one. Some infectious-diseases experts say that because viruses thrive in moist, warm settings, damp toothbrush bristles can become a hotbed for viral replication, and could infect a family member who comes in contact with the brush. Theoretically, you could even reinfect yourself, although you should have a grace period of several weeks or months when you have some natural resistance to the virus that has just left you under the weather.

Other Avenues to Cold Comfort

- Don't share eating utensils, drinking glasses, and towels with family members when there's a cold circulating through the house. Avoid leaving used towels and washcloths draped over towel hangers in the bathroom.

- When you blow your nose or sneeze, use a clean facial tissue and then dispose of it immediately. Wash your hands afterward, and empty wastebaskets frequently.

- Whenever possible, choose tissues over cloth handkerchiefs during cold and flu season. A handkerchief tucked into your pocket or purse can become a breeding ground for replicating viruses, which can then be transferred to your hands each time you touch it.

- Clean bathroom and kitchen surfaces frequently with a disinfectant that kills viruses (for example, Pine-Sol or Lysol). Do the same with telephones, light switches, doorknobs, remote control devices, and children's toys. Clean items and surfaces at your workplace in the same way.

- Sometimes the skin on the outer edges of the nostrils can become red, inflamed, and chapped because of the continuous dripping of secretions and the repeated blowing and wiping of your nose. To relieve this "red nose syndrome," apply a thin layer of petroleum jelly or skin lotion. Because you might wipe some of this lubricant away with tissue each time you blow your nose, you may have to reapply it several times during the day. Be sure to place some on the affected part of your nose just before going to sleep, so it can do its work throughout the night while you're sleeping.

· When you check the temperature of a sick family member (or yourself), disinfect the thermometer with rubbing alcohol after you use it.

· Show extra care in public rest rooms. Wash your hands thoroughly before leaving the bathroom. Once your hands are clean, use a paper towel when touching faucet knobs and exit doors.

Becoming Airborne with a Cold?

When you're struggling with a cold, you're better off avoiding airplanes. But if you have to make a trip, at least your runny nose and cough won't become worse in the air—although your ears may never forgive you. Nasal membrane swelling associated with a cold can block the eustachian tube (the channel between the nose and the middle ear). This tube normally equalizes pressure in the middle ear with the outside pressure, but when it becomes obstructed and you're in a descending airplane, the high pressure outside the ear can cause abnormal distortions and stretching of the eardrum. The result: severe pain.

If you're unable to postpone your flight during a cold, here are a few techniques to try:

· Try opening the blocked eustachian tube by swallowing and yawning. This doesn't always work when you have a cold, however.

· Use an oral or nasal-spray decongestant about an

hour prior to takeoff, and again an hour before the plane starts its descent; this medication will shrink swollen membranes, and may temporarily open blocked tubes. Chewing gum might also help.

8

A Medicine Chest for Your Cold

"If you treat a cold aggressively, you'll get over it in a week. If you don't treat it at all, it will clear up in seven days." There's more truth to that statement than most pharmaceutical companies would like to admit. Although drugstore shelves are jammed with hundreds of cold and flu remedies, here are the cold, cruel facts: These medications *cannot* cure your cold. They may relieve your symptoms, but your body's own immune system will resolve the infection in a week to ten days, and will finally vanquish the virus more effectively than any drug can.

Nevertheless, when your nose is running like a faucet and you're coughing so hard that you can barely catch your breath, you'll probably grab and gobble down just about anything that your pharmacy shelves offer for symptom relief. Each year, Americans spend over *two billion dollars* on over-the-counter cold remedies, plus many millions more on prescription drugs.

The cold remedies described in this chapter have an important advantage, and that's having withstood the scrutiny of the Food and Drug Administration and won the right to enter the marketplace. Unlike many of the treatments you read about earlier—from herbs to homeopathy—these OTC products have undergone extensive safety and efficacy testing.

If you want to try a cold or flu medication, how do you choose? The best approach is to look for a product whose ingredients blast away at the particular symptoms that you have. If you're all clogged up, you might choose a decongestant that unplugs your nose. If you have a cough that makes your chest feel as if it's ready to burst, then a cough suppressant makes sense. If you have minor aches and pains, an analgesic may give you a new lease on life. Some products contain a combination of ingredients, attacking multiple symptoms with a double- or triple-barreled assault.

Get the point? Label-reading may not be something you're eager to do when your respiratory tract is in a meltdown mode, but it's worth the effort. In the rest of this chapter, we'll help you negotiate through the maze of products out there, and help you match your symptom to the drugs most likely to help.

NASAL CONGESTION

For temporary relief of a stuffy nose, over-the-counter (OTC) decongestants are your best weapon. They shrink swollen blood vessels, reduce blood flow to the region, and open up your nasal passages, making breathing easier. As you scan the aisles of your pharmacy, you'll have to make a choice between topical and oral formulations.

Topical Decongestants

These are administered in sprays or drops. They are not only effective, but they also work quickly; the drug floods the nose—right where it can do the most good—and thus you experience its benefits within minutes. Topical decongestants also tend to have fewer side effects than the oral preparations (although they occasionally irritate the nasal tissues, causing burning, stinging or dryness), and they don't have the stimulant effects associated with oral drugs.

Examples of topical decongestants include Afrin Nasal Spray and Neo-Synephrine Maximum Strength 12 Hour Nasal Spray, both with the active ingredient *oxymetazoline*. Other sprays are available with different ingredients, including *phenylephrine* (Vicks Sinex Nasal Spray) and *xylometazoline* (Otrivin Nasal Spray).

Before using a spray, blow your nose gently to clear away as much mucus as possible. Then place the tip of the sprayer into one of your nostrils and inhale as you squeeze the container; follow the label instructions regarding the number of squirts per nostril. Don't share the sprayer with anyone else, since it may harbor cold viruses that it comes into contact with.

There are a few noteworthy concerns regarding topical products: Do not use them for more than three days, or you'll run the risk of a rebound effect and an actual worsening of your congestion; if symptoms persist beyond just a few days, begin using an oral preparation instead. Also, if you're taking MAO (monoamine oxidase) inhibitors for depression, talk to your doctor before taking decongestants (topical or oral), since the interactions can be severe in some cases.

Risk-Free Sprays

When your congestion has you feeling as though a clothespin is pinching your nostrils shut, one type of nasal spray could help—without the risk of side effects or a rebound effect. It is a saline spray that can be purchased in over-the-counter formulations with brand names such as Ocean Nasal Mist or NaSal Moisturizer AF. Or if you'd like, you can make your own saline solution: Add ¼ teaspoon of salt to 8 ounces of water and apply this mixture with a bulb syringe. You can use the commercial or do-it-yourself sprays whenever your nasal passages feel dry and congested.

Oral Decongestants

Available as pills, these include products such as Sudafed Nasal Decongestant Tablets, whose active ingredient is *pseudoephedrine*. Side effects can occur with oral formulations, including dizziness, sleep disruptions, nervousness, a racing heart, and increases in blood pressure. Oral decongestants can also slow the urine flow in men who have an enlarged prostate (benign prostatic hyperplasia). However, they do not cause the rebound effect seen with the topical decongestants, and their actions may last longer.

Before taking oral decongestants, talk to your doctor if you have very high blood pressure, glaucoma, diabetes, an enlarged prostate, or an overactive thyroid.

Time-Release Formulations: Do They Make Sense?

When you have to take medication on a regular schedule—a pill every four hours, for example—it's sometimes easy to lose track of when you should take the next tablet. For the busy and forgetful among us, time-release pills (sometimes called *extended-release* or *sustained-release*) may be the answer. Take one in the morning, and the tablet itself will automatically release modest but continuing doses throughout the day, providing ongoing symptom relief.

Several decongestants are available in the time-release format, and can provide dosing for 8-, 12-, and 24-hour periods. In some cases, their exterior coating begins to dissolve as soon as they reach the stomach, and then subsequent inner layers dissolve later in the day. Other formulations are composed of many tiny pills, which dissolve at different intervals during the day, thus keeping you well medicated at all times, including during your eight hours of sleep.

Some doctors discourage the use of timed-release decongestants, because of their concern of side effects. If you take a 24-hour formulation, for example, and begin to experience negative effects such as irritability or restlessness right away, they're concerned that you'll have to cope with those adverse symptoms until all of the drug's active ingredients are released and wear off.

Decongestants

Active Ingredients and Representative Brand Products

TOPICAL DECONGESTANTS

Naphazoline	Privine
Oxymetazoline	Afrin Nasal Spray, Duration 12 Hour Nasal Spray, Neo-Synephrine Maximum Strength 12 Hour Nasal Spray, 12 Hour Nostrilla
Phenylephrine	Vicks Sinex Nasal Spray
Xylometazoline	Otrivin Nasal Spray

ORAL DECONGESTANTS

Pseudoephedrine	Sudafed Nasal Decongestant Tablets, Triaminic AM Decongestant Formula, Efidac/24

COUGHS

Colds and coughs sometimes seem as inseparable as Bogie and Bacall. In the first day or two of sniffling and sneezing, your postnasal drip may begin to trigger a dry, hacking cough that can turn into a ''productive,'' phlegm-producing one. Those phlegmy coughs sound and feel rather brutal, but they're actually signs that the cold is resolving itself, and thus you probably don't want to do anything to muffle them. In fact, if those mucus-filled secretions aren't expelled by coughing, you could be setting yourself up for complications, particularly the spread of the infection to other parts of the respiratory tract, thus causing bronchitis or a lung infection.

Nevertheless, nothing can win more icy stares at a crowded movie theater than a cough that drowns out every key piece of dialogue on the screen. Fortunately, dozens of cough medicines are on the market, designed to take that annoying, hacking bark out of a cold. Some come as tablets, but if they aren't to your liking, you can try a syrupy formulation. If syrups don't do the job, try lozenges. Here's a closer look at what you'll find on the shelves.

Cough Suppressants

Suppressants (also called *antitussives*) do exactly what their name suggests; they work directly on the cough center in the brain, expanding the threshold that must be reached before you begin to cough. They're good for coughs that aren't doing much—that is, dry coughs that are not expelling any mucus. Remember, you don't want to suppress coughs that are bringing up phlegm; you want to suppress only dry coughs. Suppressants are the perfect choice for a dry cough that is making you uncomfortable and miserable and is ruining all hopes of a good night's sleep.

These suppressants fall into three major categories, according to their active ingredient:

- *Dextromethorphan* is a synthetic derivative of morphine, and is the most popular of the available OTC suppressants. It is found in products such as Robitussin Maximum Strength Cough Suppressant, Benylin Adult Formula Cough Suppressant, and Drixoral Cough Liquid Caps. Most doctors consider them safe and effective. Their benefits usually begin within minutes, and depending on the product, they can last about four to eight hours per dose. Side effects are uncommon (although many people insist that the taste of some products is so unpleasant that they'd prefer to deal with the cough!).

- *Diphenhydramine* is an antihistamine that can dry up the mucus in the throat and suppress coughs. Its primary side effects are related to the central nervous system, and include sleepiness or grogginess. As a result, don't take these drugs if you need to be alert (for example, to drive a car or operate heavy machinery). In fact, diphenhydramine is the active ingredient in OTC sleep aids such as Nytol Quick Caps Caplets, so its ability to cause a few yawns isn't surprising.

- *Codeine* is available as an over-the-counter cough preparation only in certain states. Though it can suppress a cough, it can also cause side effects such as constipation, an upset stomach, and sleepiness. When you take a cough medicine with codeine in it, do not use alcohol or sedatives at the same time.

Expectorants

At times, phlegm seems quite content staying just where it is, hiding out in the airways. But as part of your recovery process from a cold, you need to get it out. Expectorants are not designed to suppress coughs, but rather to loosen and thin this sputum and make it easier to cough up. The active ingredient in all expectorants is called *guaifenesin*—it's the only OTC ingredient approved for use as an expectorant. Doctors debate just how effective these expectorants are; some say that just drinking plenty of fluids—from hot tea to chicken soup—can thin mucus just as well as guaifenesin.

Cough Drops

Put a cough drop in your mouth, and it will stimulate the production of saliva, which in turn will keep your throat damp and minimize the urge to cough. Some cough drops contain topical anesthetics (such as *dyclonine*). The active ingredient in others is the suppressant *dextromethorphan*, or aromatics such as menthol, eucalyptus or peppermint oil. There are even cough drops with *hexylresorcinol*, which is primarily a bacteria-fighter, and thus won't pack a punch against the viral microorganisms that cause colds. Cough drops also often contain sugar or another sweetener to make them palatable to the taste buds. Although none of these ingredients produces much in the way of side effects, some people do experience an upset stomach when they use aromatics.

Should You Try a Chest Rub?

When you were a kid, your mother may have rubbed ointment on your chest to relieve your coughing. One of the most popular products for this use, Vicks VapoRub, contains camphor, menthol, and eucalyptus oil; another product, Mentholatum Cherry Chest Rub for Kids, is composed of camphor, natural menthol, and eucalyptus oil. If you rub a thick layer of this cream on your child's bare chest, its vapors will rise to the nose and mouth, and may help quiet a cough and help her breathe easier while she sleeps.

Cough Medicines

Active Ingredients and Representative Brand Products

COUGH SUPPRESSANTS

Dextromethorphan	Benylin Adult Formula Cough Suppressant, Drixoral Cough Liquid Caps, Pertussin Adult Extra Strength, Robitussin Maximum Strength Cough Suppressant, Robitussin Pediatric Cough Suppressant, Vicks 44 Cough Relief

| Diphenhydramine | Nytol Quick Caps Caplets, Maximum Strength Unisom Sleepgels |

EXPECTORANTS

| Guaifenesin | Benylin Expectorant, Robitussin |

COUGH DROPS/LOZENGES

Dyclonine	Sucrets Maximum Strength Wintergreen
Dextromethorphan	Sucrets 4 Hour Cough Suppressant
Menthol	Cepacol Sore Throat Lozenges, Celestial Seasonings Soothers Herbal Throat Drops, Vicks Chloraseptic Cough & Throat Drops
Hexylresorcinol	Sucrets Regular Strength Original Mint

SORE THROATS

When your throat feels like sandpaper, and the mere act of swallowing provokes screams for mercy, there are several routes to salvation. Browse through a drugstore and you'll find topical throat sprays, lozenges, and gargles that you can buy without a prescription. Yes, they can soothe and numb the nerve endings in the throat, and thus relieve minor sore throat irritation and pain; however, they can't cure the infection.

A sore throat is sometimes the first symptom of a cold, and an indication that the cold virus is running rampant in the respiratory tract, inflaming the mucous membranes. The nonprescription drugs for sore throats are mild anesthetics, and while they are often effective, their benefits are sometimes only short-lived.

Dyclonine, one of the most commonly used ingredients, is found in products such as Sucrets Maximum Strength lozenges; it is safe, and when delivered in a lozenge, its effects can last for several hours, making it a particularly effective agent. In other forms (sprays and gargles), it can provide relief for an hour or less. As with all medications, read and adhere to dosage instructions carefully.

Benzocaine, another popular ingredient, is chemically related to novocaine, the drug used by dentists. Both drugs numb nerve endings and pain. *Phenol* also deadens nerves for short periods of time.

As an adjunct to throat sprays and lozenges, an analgesic such as aspirin can further take the edge off the pain. Interestingly, you can also find relief just by sucking on simple hard candy, which will stimulate saliva production and keep the mucous membranes in the throat from becoming dry. You can also try gargling with a saltwater mixture.

There are other steps you can take to ease your throat pain. If you smoke, stop. Avoid spicy foods until the discomfort subsides. Reduce the amount of talking that you normally do. Drink hot tea and broth. If the pain becomes severe, and there are spots of pus in the back of the throat, see your doctor; you could have strep throat, which is caused by a bacterial infection, and you'll need treatment with antibiotics.

Sore Throat Medications

Active Ingredients and Representative Brand Products

Benzocaine	Lozenges: Cepacol Maximum Strength Sore Throat Lozenges, Vicks Chloraseptic Sore Throat Lozenges
Dyclonine	Lozenges: Sucrets Maximum Strength Wintergreen; sprays: Cepacol Maximum Strength Sore Throat Spray
Hexylresorcinol	Lozenges: Listerine Maximum Strength throat lozenges, Sucrets Regular Strength/Original Mints
Menthol	Lozenges: N'ICE, Halls Plus
Phenol	Lozenges: Cepastat Cherry Flavor Sore Throat Lozenges

WHAT ROLE FOR ANTIHISTAMINES?

Antihistamines are best known as allergy fighters. As their name suggests, they block the activity of histamine, the chemical your body produces when you're in the presence of allergens (pollen, mold, dust). Thus, they can relieve allergy (hay fever) symptoms such as a runny or stuffy nose.

Somehow, antihistamines (such as *chlorpheniramine, brompheniramine*, and *diphenhydramine*) have also found their way into some OTC cold medications (Comtrex, Dimetapp, TheraFlu), even though histamine is not a player in the common cold (remember, colds are caused by viruses). The allergy-like symptoms that occur with colds and flus have nothing to do with histamine—and thus they probably cannot be influenced by antihistamines. At least that's what most doctors think.

However, an occasional study is kinder to antihistamines. A recent one at the University of Virginia found that when cold sufferers took an antihistamine called *clemastine fumarate* (found in the allergy medications Tavist-1 and Tavist-D), they sneezed about 50 percent less frequently, and their mucus production was 35 percent less than that of a control group who took placebos. Other studies, however, have suggested that in cold sufferers, antihistamines may actually *thicken* mucus, and make it more difficult to expel.

No matter what the final verdict, the side effects associated with antihistamines—primarily drowsiness and decreased mental alertness—can be problematic for many people. Ironically, however, these sedative properties have been promoted as a positive component of antihistamine-containing "nighttime" cold and flu formulations such as Vicks NyQuil and TheraFlu Maximum Strength Nighttime Flu Medicine; pharmaceutical companies often advertise products like these as helping you sleep through the night. Antihistamines are incorporated into many combination cold medications and are found in some cough suppressants.

Antihistamine Cold Medications

Representative Products
Alka-Seltzer Plus Cold & Cough Medicine
Comtrex Maximum Strength Multi-Symptom
  Cold Reliever
Dimetapp Tablets
Sine-Off Sinus Medicine Caplets
TheraFlu Maximum Strength Nighttime Flu
  Medicine
Vicks NyQuil

ACHES AND PAINS

When the flu or a cold has wracked your body with muscle aches and pains, or if you're on fire with a fever that seems about ready to burst the thermometer, turn to an analgesic such as the most popular ones described here.

- *Aspirin* has been the workhorse of pain relievers for decades; in fact, although modern aspirin was first introduced in 1899, its active ingredient (salicylate) has been used by health-care practitioners for virtually thousands of years. Aspirin is the least expensive painkiller you can find, particularly in its generic versions. Its acidic properties make some people prone to stomach irritation when taking it. Aspirin can also trigger intestinal bleeding, particularly with long-term use. A small percentage of individuals (especially people with asthma) are allergic to aspirin.

- *Ibuprofen* (Advil, Nuprin, Motrin) is another effective pain reliever and is less likely to cause the irritation and bleeding associated with aspirin (although it is not immune to these problems). Some people develop allergic skin rashes associated with ibuprofen use. With both aspirin and ibuprofen, you should eat something before swallowing the pills.
- *Acetaminophen* is best known by the trade name Tylenol. It poses much less risk of side effects and allergic reactions than other analgesics.

All of these medications are capable of reducing a fever associated with colds and flu (although for a low-grade fever, you may be better off just letting the fever do its infection-fighting job). None, however, should be taken in excess. Also, keep in mind that these OTC drugs aren't going to relieve your runny nose or sore throat. In fact, here's the catch associated with painkillers: Research shows that they may actually *interfere* with the activity of the immune system, and thus may prolong or worsen your cold symptoms. One study found more nasal congestion and a decreased immune response in people with colds who had taken aspirin or acetaminophen. More research is needed, but for now, use analgesics only when you need them.

Remember, these drugs are safe when taken in the dosages prescribed on the labels. For children, however, there could be serious risks associated with aspirin use. Aspirin has been linked to a rare, serious, and sometimes life-threatening illness called Reye's syndrome, which can cause injuries to the brain, the liver, and other organs. Here's a hard-and-fast rule: If your child or teenager has a fever, or other flu or chicken pox symptoms, do *not* give him aspirin. Acetaminophen is a much better choice, and will be just as effective in bringing down his temperature.

WHAT ABOUT A "SHOTGUN" DRUG?

When you're coping with the Mother of All Colds, treating it with only one medication may seem like the equivalent of managing cancer with an aspirin. Enter the world of combination or ''shotgun'' medications such as Contac Severe Cold and Flu Caplets and Robitussin Cough & Cold Liqui-Gels.

Some combination drugs have two or three ingredients; others have as many as six. Most combination cold remedies contain a decongestant; many also have an antihistamine, an aspirin (or acetaminophen), and a cough suppressant and/or expectorant. Some even have alcohol in them.

Many doctors believe that these shotgun drugs are a

classic case of overkill. As we've already pointed out, you should choose cold-medication ingredients that target your particular symptoms. The combination drugs frequently give you more than you need, and eliminate any chance to adjust dosages as your symptoms wax or wane.

To confuse matters, it simply makes no sense to take a medication containing *both* a cough suppressant and an expectorant. After all, the expectorant is supposed to loosen the phlegm so you can cough it up; but the suppressant is intended to interfere with the cough reflex and quiet a cough. And when an antihistamine is included in the formulation as well, presumably to dry up mucus, isn't it counterproductive to combine it with an expectorant, which moistens and loosens the mucus so it can be expelled?

If you're thinking about trying a combination drug (some of the most popular, and their ingredients, are listed in the adjoining box), keep in mind that they tend to be more costly than a single-ingredient product, and they may not give you the precise medications you need.

What Are You Really Getting with Combination Medications?

When you purchase a combination medication, it might include everything you need to control your cold symptoms—and more. To help you determine what you're getting, here are the ingredients in some of the more popular "shotgun" cold drugs.

Advil Cold & Sinus Caplets and Tablets
Pseudoephedrine (decongestant)
Ibuprofen (analgesic)

Alka-Seltzer Plus Cold and Cough Medicine
Phenylpropanolamine (decongestant)
Dextromethorphan (cough suppressant)
Chlorpheniramine (antihistamine)
Aspirin (analgesic)

Benadryl Allergy/Cold Tablets
Pseudoephedrine (decongestant)
Diphenhydramine (antihistamine)
Acetaminophen (analgesic)

Cheracol Plus Multi-Symptom Cough/Cold Formula
Phenylpropanolamine (decongestant)
Dextromethorphan (cough suppressant)
Chlorpheniramine (antihistamine)
Alcohol

Comtrex Multi-Symptom Cold Reliever Tablets
Pseudoephedrine (decongestant)
Dextromethorphan (cough suppressant)
Chlorpheniramine (antihistamine)
Acetaminophen (analgesic)

Contac Severe Cold and Flu Caplets
Phenylpropanolamine (decongestant)
Dextromethorphan (cough suppressant)

Chlorpheniramine (antihistamine)
Acetaminophen (analgesic)

Dimetapp Cold & Cough Liqui-Gels
Phenylpropanolamine (decongestant)
Brompheniramine (antihistamine)
Dextromethorphan (cough suppressant)

Drixoral Cold & Flu Extended-Release Tablets
Pseudoephedrine (decongestant)
Dexbrompheniramine (antihistamine)
Acetaminophen (analgesic)

Robitussin Cold & Cough Liqui-Gels
Pseudoephedrine (decongestant)
Dextromethorphan (cough suppressant)
Guaifenesin (expectorant)

Sinarest Tablets
Pseudoephedrine (decongestant)
Chlorpheniramine (antihistamine)
Acetaminophen (analgesic)

Sudafed Severe Cold Formula Tablets
Pseudoephedrine (decongestant)
Dextromethorphan (cough suppressant)
Acetaminophen (analgesic)

TheraFlu Maximum Strength Nighttime Flu, Cold & Cough Medicine
Pseudoephedrine (decongestant)
Dextromethorphan (cough suppressant)

Acetaminophen (analgesic)
Chlorpheniramine (antihistamine)

Triaminic Expectorant

Phenylpropanolamine (decongestant)
Guaifenesin (expectorant)

9

What's in Your Doctor's Black Bag?

As you've already read, there's a lot you can do on your own to prevent and treat colds and flus, using the OTC medications available in the pharmacy along with a growing array of alternative approaches. As a result, you must be wondering whether your own physician has been left out of the loop entirely, with little to suggest beyond those strategies you can pursue on your own.

However, don't overlook your doctor as part of the mix. Particularly when it comes to the flu vaccine, or to prescribing drugs to treat complications associated with life's most common illnesses, your doctor can round out a program that increases your odds of staying as healthy as possible throughout the cold and flu season.

Of course, a runny nose and a cough generally aren't anything to be overly concerned about. In a week or so, the symptoms will run their course, and were it not for a wastebasket full of used tissue nearby, there might be no reminders at all of the onslaught of sneezing that disrupted your life.

On occasion, however, colds run a stubborn course that deviates from the norm. Your dry, hacking cough may become productive with green phlegm and start setting volcanic records for its earthshaking uproar. Your low-grade fever might start climbing up the thermometer, and you could suddenly feel as if a three-alarm fire is burning inside of you. Your ears may start to throb, you could have trouble breathing, and your chest might begin to ache. That's the time to see your doctor to make sure that your simple cold and cough aren't something much more serious, like pneumonia.

THE ANTIBIOTIC ARSENAL

Antibiotics and colds? There couldn't be a more imperfect match. After all, even though antibiotics can often wipe out bacterial infections with ease, they are virtually useless in the face of viral illnesses, including colds and flus.

Nevertheless, physicians have had a love affair with antibiotics for decades, and patients have joined in the romance, feeling that a doctor's visit is wasted if they haven't left with a prescription in their hand. Here are the cold facts: Antibiotics are prescribed in the majority of cases where patients need deliverance from a viral respiratory illness. In a 1996 study at the University of Kentucky, Lexington, researchers found that 60 percent of patients seen in doctors' offices or emergency rooms for the common cold were prescribed an antibiotic. A year later, University of Colorado researchers arrived at a similar conclusion; they found that in 50 to 70 percent of cases in which patients saw their doctors for colds or other upper respiratory infections, antibiotics were prescribed.

No wonder many infectious-diseases experts are concerned that antibiotics are being overused, exacting a heavy price that we're all beginning to feel. Specifically, when antibiotics are used too often, bacteria develop resistance to them, thus sometimes rendering these drugs ineffective when confronted with a serious bacterial infection such as pneumonia or meningitis. The problem of resistance is becoming more worrisome year by year.

There are times, however, when the use of antibiotics does make sense for respiratory infections. If your doctor has determined that you've developed a bacterial complication—such as an ear or sinus infection—then she should write a prescription faster than you can say "penicillin."

Do You Have Complications?

When your symptoms simply won't go away, you might have more than a simple cold. The inflammation could have moved down the breathing tubes and begun creating havoc within your respiratory tract. Bacterial complications can affect the throat (strep throat), the ears (otitis media), the air passages to the lungs (bronchitis) and the lungs themselves (pneumonia). Here are some signs that could indicate a secondary infection. Any of these symptoms should warrant a trip to the doctor's office:

- Increases in mucus production, typically colored green, gray, or dark yellow; blood in the phlegm
- A high fever (above 101 degrees) for more than two to three days
- Mild to severe pain or pressure around the eyes, in an ear, and/or in the cheeks or upper teeth
- Hoarseness
- Swollen glands in the neck
- A severe sore throat, with pus in the throat and difficulty swallowing
- Pain in the upper chest that worsens when you cough
- A severe, hacking cough
- Shortness of breath
- Persistent wheezing

FIGHTING FLU: A SHOT IN THE ARM

One of the best ways to minimize your risk of complications and increase your chances of breezing through the influenza season without a cough is to get a flu shot every year. Public-health officials believe that certain people *need* annual flu vaccines, such as the elderly and those with certain chronic illnesses (see the box on page 156). But frankly, anyone who'd like to avoid being incapacitated for a few days by a flu attack would be wise to roll up his or her sleeve and get a shot. Studies indicate that the vaccine is 70 to 85 percent effective in preventing influenza, although it is a little less effective in the elderly and the chronically ill. However, even when the vaccine doesn't prevent the flu altogether, it minimizes the severity of flu symptoms.

Infectious-diseases specialist Steven Mostow, M.D., tells his patients that the best time to get the vaccine is between mid-October and mid-November each year. This gives your body enough time to build up infection-fighting antibodies before the flu bug unleashes its fury, typically beginning in December; it takes two to four weeks for these antibodies to fully develop.

By the way, even if you got a flu shot last year, you need another one for the upcoming flu season. That's because the composition of the vaccine changes annually to protect against the specific flu subtypes that are expected to dominate in the upcoming fall and winter. Flu viruses are able to mutate, or change themselves, and thus researchers worldwide must constantly monitor the evolution of these viruses. For example, the strains showing up in the Southern Hemisphere one flu season may be transported to North America during the next season. Each January, members of an FDA advisory committee meet to determine which subtypes of the flu virus will be made part of the vaccine for the following flu season.

Although some people believe that the flu vaccine is risky, side effects are rare. The most likely reaction is redness or soreness at the site of the injection, which usually will last no more than two days. The flu shot is made from killed or inactivated virus, and thus cannot give you the flu.

Are You in a High-Risk Group?

Should you get a flu shot this year? According to the Centers for Disease Control and Prevention, anyone 6 months of age or older who runs the risk of influenza complications should be vaccinated. If you fall into any of the following categories, you are a prime candidate for the vaccine:

- Older individuals (age 65 and over)
- Residents of nursing homes or other long-term care facilities
- People with chronic heart, lung, or kidney disease
- Individuals with diabetes, asthma, or anemia
- People whose immune systems are compromised (due to AIDS, cancer treatment, or long-term corticosteroid use)
- Children and teenagers who are receiving long-term aspirin therapy and would be at risk for developing Reye's syndrome if they caught the flu
- Women who will be 6 months pregnant or more during the flu season, or who will have just delivered a baby
- People who care for others at high risk for the flu (for example doctors and nurses), or individuals (such as family members) who live with those at risk

Some people should *avoid* flu shots, primarily those who are allergic to eggs (the vaccines are prepared with viruses injected into fertilized hens' eggs, where they reproduce before finally being made noninfectious in the lab with a formaldehyde solution). Also, if you're running a high fever, wait until it subsides before being vaccinated.

Good News for Needle-Phobics

"I'd get a flu shot, but I'm terrified of needles." Sound familiar? Many people will do just about anything to avoid being vaccinated, including accepting the risk of catching the flu bug. But tests are underway on new influenza vaccines that could relegate the needles used for flu-prevention injections into the Smithsonian. Vaccines are being developed that would provide protection via a nasal spray or nose drops. Other research is aimed at developing a pill that could prevent the flu by keeping the virus from attaching itself to human cells.

In 1997, investigators conducting a study funded by the National Institute of Allergy and Infectious Diseases reported that when the flu vaccine was administered to young children as a nasal spray, it was safe and produced good antibody response. Most important, it provided protection against the flu in 93 percent of cases. If subsequent studies also show positive results, researchers predict that the new nasal-spray/nose-drop formulations could be on the market as early as 1999.

By the way, another nasal spray—this one to treat the common cold—is being studied as well. In research published in the *Annals of Internal Medicine* in 1996, part of a group of 411 people (ages 14 to 56) with newly symptomatic colds were given a spray containing a medication called ipratropium, while others got a placebo. After four days, those receiving the drug (two squirts per nostril, three to four times a day) had experienced a 20 to 30 percent decrease in their sneezing and nasal discharge, compared to the placebo group, but there was no difference in their nasal congestion. (Ipratropium is already on the market, approved for use in allergy patients, and is available as a nasal spray under the brand name Atrovent).

A DRUG FOR THE FLU

So you forgot to get an influenza shot, or just couldn't bear to subject yourself to an injection. You just kept putting it off—and then the flu struck. What now?

You can react like most people—get into bed and cope as best you can until the fever, chills, and drippy nose run their course. Or you can call your doctor and ask for a little help from his prescription pad.

There are two little-known oral antiviral drugs that might be able to rescue you from the onslaught of the flu, even after the virus has invaded your body and symptoms have started. These drugs—Symmetrel (amantadine) and Flumadine (rimantadine)—are effective only against the influenza A virus (the most prevalent form), but if you take them early in the course of the illness, you might be able to cut into your misery index and stop the flu in its tracks. Studies show that when these medications are taken within 24 to 48 hours of the appearance of symptoms, they can decrease fevers and reduce the length of the illness by about one-third, getting you back on your feet a lot sooner. Also, if your community is in the middle of a flu epidemic, and you never got a flu shot, you can use these drugs prophylactically; taken daily, for a period of weeks or even months, they can protect against catching the flu in about 70 to 80 percent of cases.

Symmetrel and Flumadine can be taken by otherwise healthy adults and children over the age of 1. Side effects? A small percentage of people have reported feeling dizzy or nauseated or have experienced disrupted sleep; in general, Flumadine produces fewer toxic effects than does Symmetrel.

AUTHOR'S NOTE

If you've been reading this book while sniffling and sneezing, anyone within earshot of your symptoms and suffering may have rushed to your aid with a tissue and the words, "God bless you." As comforting as that statement may be, divine intervention is unlikely, and you'll probably have to deal with your illness as best you can.

In this book, you've learned strategies that can give you an upper hand in your battle to prevent and manage the common cold and influenza. Some of the steps—from frequent hand washing to high doses of vitamin C—may have been familiar to you for years. Others, including the use of echinacea, zinc lozenges, and homeopathy, may be new, but can quickly become part of your overall disease-fighting plan.

Perhaps the best news of all is that colds and flus are self-limiting illnesses. Unless complications develop, they'll certainly make you uncomfortable for several days, and perhaps force you to miss work for a while, but they aren't life-threatening. There are still no miracle

cures to deliver you from the common cold, and none
are on the horizon. But from chicken soup to Chinese
medicine, there's a lot you can do to loosen the grip of
the cold and flu viruses, and allow yourself to live more
cold-free than you may have thought possible.

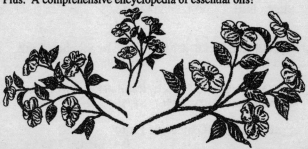